KEY TOPICS IN

GASTROENTEROLOGY

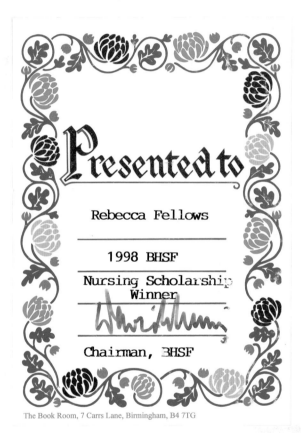

Presented to

Rebecca Fellows

1998 BHSF

Nursing Scholarship
Winner

Chairman, BHSF

The Book Room, 7 Carrs Lane, Birmingham, B4 7TG

The KEY TOPICS Series

Advisors:

T.M. Craft *Department of Anaesthesia and Intensive Care, Royal United Hospital, Bath, UK*
C.S. Garrard *Intensive Therapy Unit, John Radcliffe Hospital, Oxford, UK*
P.M. Upton *Department of Anaesthetics, Royal Cornwall Hospital, Truro, UK*

Anaesthesia, Second Edition

Obstetrics and Gynaecology, Second Edition

Accident and Emergency Medicine

Paediatrics, Second Edition

Orthopaedic Surgery

Otolaryngology

Ophthalmology

Psychiatry

General Surgery

Renal Medicine

Trauma

Chronic Pain

Oral and Maxillofacial Surgery

Oncology

Cardiovascular Medicine

Neurology

Neonatology

Gastroenterology

Forthcoming titles include:
Respiratory Medicine

Thoracic Surgery

Critical Care

Orthopaedic Trauma Surgery

Accident and Emergency Medicine, Second Edition

KEY TOPICS IN
GASTROENTEROLOGY

SIMON H.C. ANDERSON
MRCP
*Specialist Registrar in Gastroenterology, King's College Hospital,
London, UK*

GARETH DAVIES
MD MRCP
*Consultant Gastroenterologist, Harrogate District Hospital,
Harrogate, UK*

HARRY R. DALTON
BSc DPhil FRCP Dip. Med. Ed.
*Consultant Gastroenterologist, Royal Cornwall Hospital, Truro
and Honorary Senior Lecturer, University of Plymouth, Plymouth, UK*

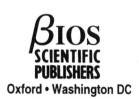

*β*IOS
**SCIENTIFIC
PUBLISHERS**
Oxford • Washington DC

First published 1999

A CIP catalogue record for this book is available from the British Library.

ISBN 1 85996 281 5

BIOS Scientific Publishers Ltd
9 Newtec Place, Magdalen Road, Oxford OX4 1RE, UK
Tel. +44 (0)1865 726286. Fax. +44 (0)1865 246823
World Wide Web home page: http://www.bios.co.uk/

Important Note from the Publisher
The information contained within this book was obtained by BIOS Scientific Publishers Ltd from sources believed by us to be reliable. However, while every effort has been made to ensure its accuracy, no responsibility for loss or injury whatsoever occasioned to any person acting or refraining from action as a result of information contained herein can be accepted by the authors or publishers.

The reader should remember that medicine is a constantly evolving science and while the authors and publishers have ensured that all dosages, applications and practices are based on current indications, there may be specific practices which differ between communities. You should always follow the guidelines laid down by the manufacturers of specific products and the relevant authorities in the country in which you are practising.

Production Editor: Jonathan Gunning.
Typeset by J&L Composition Ltd, Filey, UK.
Printed by T.J. International Ltd, Padstow, UK.

CONTENTS

ABBREVIATIONS

5-ASA	5-aminosalicylic acid
5-HIAA	5-hydroxyindoleacetic acid
5-HT	5-hydroxytryptamine
5FU	5-fluorouracil
AFP	alpha-fetoprotein
AIDS	acquired immune deficiency syndrome
ALF	acute liver failure
ALP	alkaline phosphatase
ALT	alanine transaminase
AMA	anti-mitochondrial antibodies
APC	adenomatous polyposis coli
AST	aspartate aminotransferase
AZT	azothymidine
BNF	British National Formulary
BSG	British Society of Gastroenterology
BSP	bromsulphthalein
CAH	chronic autoimmune hepatitis
cAMP	cyclic adenosine monophosphate
CD	coeliac disease
CEA	carcinoembryonic antigen
CLO	campylobacter-like organism
CMV	cytomegalovirus
CNS	central nervous system
CRP	C-reactive protein
CSF	cerebrospinal fluid
CT	computerized tomography
ddC	dideoxycytosine
ddI	dideoxyinosine
DIC	disseminated intravascular coagulation
DNA	deoxyribonucleic acid
DU	duodenal ulcer
EBV	Epstein–Barr virus
ECG	electrocardiogram
EEG	electroencephalogram
ELAD	extracorporeal liver assist device
ELISA	enzyme-linked immunosorbent assay
ENT	ear, nose and throat
ERCP	endoscopic retrograde cholangiopancreatography
ESR	erythrocyte sedimentation rate
ESWL	extracorporeal shock wave lithotripsy
FAP	familial adenomatous polyposis
FOB	faecal occult blood
GFD	gluten-free diet
GGT	gamma glutamyl transpeptidase

GI	gastrointestinal
GM-CSF	granulocyte-macrophage colony stimulating factor
GOR	gastro-oesophageal reflux
GORD	gastro-oesophageal reflux disease
H&E	haematoxylin and eosin
HAS	human albumin solution
HAV	hepatitis A virus
HB Ab	anti-hepatitis B antibody
HBcAb	anti-hepatitis B core antibody
HBcAg	hepatitis B core antigen
HBeAb	anti-hepatitis B 'e' antibody
HBeAg	hepatitis B 'e' antigen
HBIG	hepatitis B immunoglobulin
HBsAb	anti-hepatitis B surface antibody
HBsAg	hepatitis B surface antigen
HBV	hepatitis B virus
HCC	hepatocellular carcinoma
HCV	hepatitis C virus
HDV	hepatitis D virus
HELLP	**h**aemolysis, **e**levated **l**iver enzymes, **l**ow **p**latelet count
HEV	hepatitis E virus
HGV	hepatitis G virus
HIDA	hydroxy-iminodiacetic acid
HII	hepatic iron index
HIV	human immunodeficiency virus
HLA	human leucocyte antigen
HMPAO	hexamethyl propyleneamine oxime
HNPCC	hereditary non-polyposis colorectal cancer
HSV	herpes simplex virus
HUS	haemolytic uraemic syndrome
i.m.	intramuscular
i.v.	intravenous
IBS	irritable bowel syndrome
ICP	intracranial pressure
IFN-α	interferon alpha
Ig	immunoglobulin
IL	interleukin
INR	international normalized ratio
IPSID	immunoproliferative small intestinal disease
ISG	immune serum globulin
ITU	intensive therapy unit
KS	Kaposi's sarcoma
LDH	lactate dehydrogenase
LE	lupus erythematosus
LKM	liver and kidney microsome
LOS	lower oesophageal sphincter
MAC	*Mycobacterium avium* complex

MALToma	mucosa-associated lymphoid tissue lymphoma
MCT	medium-chain triglycerides
MEN	multiple endocrine neoplasia
MHC	major histocompatability complex
MRC	magnetic resonance cholangiography
MRI	magnetic resonance imaging
MTBE	methyl-tert-butyl-ether
NBT-PABA	N-benzoyl-L-tyrosyl-p-aminobenzoic acid
Nd:YAG	neodymium-yttrium aluminium-garnet
NHL	non-Hodgkin's lymphoma
NSAID	non-steroidal anti-inflammatory drug
OGD	oesophagogastroduodenoscopy
PABA	para-amino benzoic acid
PAS	periodic acid–Schiff
PBC	primary biliary cirrhosis
PCA	patient-controlled analgesia
P_{CO_2}	partial pressure of carbon dioxide
PCR	polymerase chain reaction
PMC	pseudomembranous colitis
P_{O_2}	partial pressure of oxygen
PSC	primary sclerosing cholangitis
PT	prothrombin time
PTC	percutaneous transhepatic cholangiography
PUVA	psoralen and ultraviolet-A light
RIBA	recombinant immunoblot assay
RNA	ribonucleic acid
SBP	spontaneous bacterial peritonitis
SBT	small bowel transplantation
SeHCAT	^{75}Se-labelled homotaurocholic acid
SLE	systemic lupus erythematosus
TIPSS	transjugular intrahepatic portosystemic stent shunts
TLOR	transient lower oesophageal sphincter relaxation
TNM	tumour node metastasis classification
TPN	total parenteral nutrition
TTP	thrombotic thrombocytopenic purpura
UDCA	ursodeoxycholic acid
UGT	upper gastrointestinal tract
VIP	vasoactive intestinal peptide
WHO	World Health Organization

PREFACE

This is not a complete textbook in gastroenterology and should not be treated as such. We have tried to address the major subjects in gastroenterology in what we hope is a practical and readable manner.

Key Topics in Gastroenterology is essential reading for MRCP candidates, Senior House Officers and Junior Specialist Registrars in gastroenterology, but we hope other non-specialist doctors will also find it helpful.

We would like to thank our publishers, BIOS, particularly Jonathan Ray and Jonathan Gunning for their help, understanding and forbearance. We also thank Dr Annabel Carter for preparing the index.

Simon Anderson
Gareth Davies
Harry Dalton

ABNORMAL LIVER TESTS

Serum levels of bilirubin, and of enzymes that originate from the liver, are useful to establish the diagnosis of liver disease, monitor disease progression and plan necessary treatment. The term 'liver function tests' is technically misleading as they do not reflect the functioning capacity of the liver. The prothrombin time, and, to a lesser extent, the serum albumin, are better indicators of the synthetic function of the liver.

Bilirubin

Bilirubin is formed from the breakdown of haem (predominantly haemoglobin) in the reticuloendothelial system and, to a lesser extent, from liver cytochromes. Bilirubin is made water-soluble by conjugation with glucuronic acid to form monoglucuronides and diglucuronides. Conjugated bilirubin and the other contents of bile (e.g. bile salts) pass into the intestine. Intestinal bacteria break down conjugated bilirubin, producing stercobilinogen and stercobilin. Some stercobilinogen and stercobilin is absorbed in the distal bowel, most is then re-excreted in the bile (enterohepatic circulation); small amounts may appear in the urine, where they are termed urobilinogen and urobilin, respectively. Stercobilin (or urobilin) is pigmented, and contributes to the colour of the stool (or urine). See also 'Jaundice' (p. 180).

1. Unconjugated hyperbilirubinaemia. Under normal circumstances the percentage of total bilirubin that is unconjugated is <10%. Even with severely compromised liver function, the liver retains much of its ability to conjugate bilirubin. Thus, hyperbilirubinaemia is labelled 'unconjugated' only when >80% is in the unconjugated form. Causes of unconjugated hyperbilirubinaemia include haemolysis and Gilbert's syndrome.

2. Conjugated hyperbilirubinaemia. This arises in either cholestatic or hepatocellular disease, and is usually accompanied by a rise in liver enzymes, with alkaline phosphatase proportionately higher than transaminases.

3. Bilirubinuria. Under normal circumstances (and in cases of unconjugated hyperbilirubinaemia), bilirubin is not detected in the urine. In cholestasis, a small fraction of conjugated bilirubin is excreted in the urine, giving it a characteristically dark colour. The commercially available 'dipstix' are a sensitive test to detect conjugated bilirubin in the urine. In acute viral hepatitis, bilirubin appears in the urine before the onset of jaundice, and thus a positive 'dipstix' test may favour the diagnosis in a pre-icteric patient.

Normally, a small amount of urobilinogen is detectable in the urine, reflecting an intact enterohepatic circulation. In complete bile duct obstruction, no bilirubin is excreted into the intestine and hence urinary urobilinogen is absent. In practice this is seldom measured, as the diagnosis is usually suggested by more sensitive serum and radiological tests.

Serum aminotransferases Aminotransferases are ubiquitous enzymes involved in the conversion of amino acids to alpha-keto acids. They are found in various tissues including the liver, heart and skeletal muscle, and hence injury to any number of tissues can result in elevated levels. The two aminotransferases routinely measured are aspartate transaminase (AST) and alanine transaminase (ALT). ALT is relatively more specific for liver disease, and an elevated level almost always indicates some degree of ongoing liver injury. Liver disease is not excluded by normal levels of transaminases (advanced cirrhosis and hepatitis C being good examples of this).

In normal circumstances the AST:ALT ratio is close to 1. In those with a ratio of >2, a diagnosis of alcoholic liver disease should be considered. In those with chronically elevated aminotransferases, an ALT:AST ratio of >2 may indicate non-alcoholic steatohepatitis (fatty liver).

Some causes of elevated hepatic aminotransferases are listed in *Table 1*, but these categories are not invariable and in practice there is considerable overlap between them.

Elevated transaminases are often detected incidentally in

Table 1. Causes of abnormal hepatic aminotransferase levels

Level	Causes
Low normal (0–20 units/l)	Chronic renal failure
Mild elevation (50–400 units/l)	Chronic liver disease (viral, autoimmune, alcohol)
	Steatosis or steatohepatitis
	Acute fatty liver of pregnancy
	Extrahepatic biliary obstruction
	Drug-induced liver injury
	Passive congestion (Budd–Chiari, cardiac, veno-occlusive)
	Liver malignancy (primary or secondary)
Moderate elevation (400–2000 units/l)	Acute hepatitis (viral or autoimmune)
	Drug-induced liver injury
	Acute biliary obstruction
	Toxins
High elevation (2000–30 000 units/l)	Acute liver failure from any cause
	Shock liver (acute ischaemic injury)

'routine screens'. A reasonable checklist of common causes to exclude would be:

- Alcohol abuse (it is useful to repeat the test after a period of abstinence).
- Steatosis (usually due to obesity or diabetes).
- Chronic hepatitis (viral or autoimmune).
- Drugs.
- Haemochromatosis.
- Right heart failure.

Other causes such as Wilson's disease and α_1-antitrypsin deficiency are often searched for via blood tests, but this is probably not justified as a 'first-line' screen in patients with no other features, due to the rarity of these causes.

Alkaline phosphatase

Different isoenzymes of alkaline phosphatase (ALP) are found in various organs – principally the liver, bone, intestine and placenta; its function is unknown. In the liver, ALP is bound to the bile canalicular membrane. In conditions of cholestasis, serum ALP rises due to increased synthesis rather than impaired secretion. Serum levels elevated over four-fold strongly suggest cholestasis, whereas lesser rises may accompany any type of liver injury. Important non-hepatic causes of a raised ALP include normal adolescence and pregnancy, metastatic bone disease and Paget's disease. A concomitantly raised serum gamma glutamyl transpeptidase (GGT) or 5'-nucleotidase suggests a hepatic source. Isoenzyme analysis can help differentiate between liver and bone sources.

Possible causes of an elevated liver-isoenzyme ALP are listed in *Table 2*. Once again these categories are not invariable or diagnostic, and in practice there is a considerable overlap between the diseases in each category.

Gamma glutamyl transpeptidase

Gamma glutamyl transpeptidase (GGT), like ALP, is an enzyme of the intrahepatic biliary canaliculi. It is more sensitive to biliary obstruction than ALP, and is useful to confirm a hepatic source of a raised ALP. Causes of an elevated level of GGT are therefore also those of a raised ALP.

GGT is also elevated in any condition of hepatocellular injury, including alcohol, drugs (particularly those that induce liver enzymes) and solid tumour liver metastases. In alcohol abuse, an isolated raised GGT may be found, but more commonly other liver enzymes are raised too.

Lactate dehydrogenase

Like the aminotransferases, lactate dehydrogenase (LDH) is abundant in the liver and is released following any form of liver insult. Elevated serum levels are also found in a variety of diseases (e.g. haemolysis and neoplasia (particularly lymphomas)) and hence it is not routinely measured in liver disease.

Table 2. Causes of abnormal hepatic alkaline phosphatase levels

Level	Causes
Low normal (<150 units/l)	Hypothyroidism Wilson's disease with haemolysis
Moderate elevation (250–750 units/l) (bilirubin often normal)	Primary biliary cirrhosis Primary or secondary sclerosing cholangitis Extrahepatic biliary obstruction Hepatic malignancy (primary or secondary, including leukaemia) Infiltrations/space-occupying lesions (e.g. abscess, granulomas, amyloid, lymphomas) Acute or chronic hepatitis Chronic liver disease including cirrhosis
High elevation (>750 units/l) (bilirubin usually raised)	Primary biliary cirrhosis Sclerosing cholangitis Hepatic lymphoma Hepatic granulomatous disease (e.g. sarcoid)

Further reading

Neuschwander-Tetri BA. Common blood tests for liver disease. *Postgraduate Medicine*, 1995; **98:** 49–63.

Related topics of interest

ACHALASIA

The term 'achalasia' means failure to relax. This describes the chief abnormality of this disorder – the failure of the lower oesophageal sphincter to relax during swallowing. The other associated abnormalites are a high resting pressure of the lower oesophageal sphincter and aperistalsis of the oesophageal body.

Aetiology

The cause of achalasia is unknown, but there is some evidence to suggest a viral infection (possibly by a neurotropic herpes virus) of the myenteric (Auerbach's) plexus of the oesophagus. Pathological changes include distortion and loss of ganglion cells in the oesophageal wall and Wallerian degeneration (indicating that denervation of oesophageal smooth muscle is one of the mechanisms involved).

Clinical features

The disease may present at any age, most commonly in middle age. The sex incidence is equal. Symptoms include progressive dysphagia for both solids and liquids (in 80–100%), retrosternal chest discomfort (in 50%), weight loss, and regurgitation of undigested food, often at night (which should always suggest the diagnosis). Patients may complain of pulmonary symptoms including a nocturnal cough (which occurs in 30%) or, more rarely, features of aspiration. The average duration of symptoms is 2 years, which is a distinguishing feature from oesophageal carcinoma.

Investigations

- Chest X-ray may show an air–fluid level in the superior mediastinum, an absent gastric bubble or, rarely, a double right heart border (more typically seen in other causes of a megaoesophagus).
- Barium swallow is the screening test of choice (but does not exclude early achalasia). The barium is seen to lie in an atonic, food-filled oesophagus, which is maximally dilated at its distal portion. The lower oesophageal sphincter fails to open normally, and barium is seen to trickle through this tonic portion, producing a so-called 'bird's beak' appearance.
- Endoscopy is mandatory, particularly to exclude carcinoma. Features of uncomplicated achalasia include a food-filled, dilated oesophagus with a lower oesophageal stricture with normal mucosa. The stricture usually allows the passage of an endoscope.
- Manometric studies usually provide a definitive diagnosis. To be able to make the diagnosis there must be an absence of peristalsis in the oesophageal body. The resting pressure of the lower oesophageal sphincter is increased, typically above 30 mmHg, and the lower oesophageal sphincter usually fails to relax completely on swallowing. The

amplitude of the pressure waves decreases in the dilated oesophagus and they typically become broad-based.

Differential diagnosis

An adenocarcinoma of the cardia or gastro-oesophageal junction may produce similar clinical and radiological findings (pseudoachalasia). A duration of symptoms of less than 6 months, age greater than 50 years and marked weight loss are more suggestive of a malignancy. Endoscopy, computerized tomography (CT) scan and endoscopic ultrasound are useful at detecting occult tumours in this region. Occasionally, squamous carcinomas, oesophageal lymphomas and metastatic spread from pancreatic, prostatic and bronchial tumours can produce similar features. Other rarer causes of a megaoesophagus include systemic sclerosis, Chagas' disease (due to infection with the parasite *Trypanosomiasis cruzi*), sarcoidosis and amyloidosis.

Treatment

The aim of the various methods of treatment is to promote oesophageal emptying whilst avoiding gastro-oesophageal reflux (GOR).

1. Dilatation procedures. These procedures, using pneumatic or hydrostatic dilators under X-ray guidance, are the initial treatment of choice. Pneumatic dilators are most commonly used and a minimum diameter of dilatation of 3–4 cm is aimed for. A single dilatation produces very good results in two-thirds of patients, and repeated dilatations are effective in approximately three-quarters. The major risk is oesophageal perforation, which occurs in approximately 2% of patients. If this is suspected, an expiratory chest radiograph should be performed an hour after the procedure (looking for air in the mediastinum or a pneumothorax). A 6-hour in-hospital stay for observation is also warranted. Treatment of an oesophageal perforation is conservative in the first instance – keeping the patient nil-by-mouth, administering intravenous (i.v.) antibiotics and fluids and, in some cases, total parenteral nutrition.

2. Surgical procedures. The open or laparoscopic Heller procedure (anterior myotomy of the circular muscle layer) is the operation of choice. This is combined with an antireflux procedure, with an excellent result being obtained in 50–90% of patients. Despite this, standard antireflux therapy may be needed to control symptoms and prevent oesophageal peptic stricture formation (a recognized complication after surgery).

3. Endoscopic injection. Injection of *Clostridium botulinum* toxin into the gastro-oesophageal junction has been shown to be beneficial. It may be useful for the frail or elderly who are unable to withstand more aggressive procedures. Repeated injections may be required.

4. Medical treatments. Drugs such as nifedipine (10–20 mg orally), isosorbide dinitrate (5 mg sublingually) before each meal are used in some patients. They are thought to act by relaxing the smooth muscle in the lower oesophageal sphincter. They can also be used as adjuvantive therapy postoperatively, or in those not suitable for an operation, but results are generally disappointing.

Carcinoma risk

The incidence of oesophageal squamous carcinoma is increased in those with untreated achalasia. This complication is now rare, although earlier studies have shown incidence rates of 2–6%. Mucosal irritation due to stasis is thought to be a factor, as most carcinomas arise in those with prolonged symptoms. As such tumours arise in the dilated segment of the oesophagus, they produce few early symptoms and are usually well-advanced on presentation.

Further reading

Kadakia SC. Coping with achalasia. *Postgraduate Medicine*, 1993; **93(5):** 249–60.

Related topics of interest

Dysphagia (p. 98)
Oesophageal carcinoma (p. 215)
Oesophageal dysmotility (p. 219)

ACUTE LIVER FAILURE

Acute liver failure (ALF) is the sudden and severe impairment of liver function, characterized by the development of encephalopathy, coagulopathy and metabolic derangements, together with cardiorespiratory and renal failure. The condition is further subdivided according to the time between the onset of jaundice and the development of encephalopathy (see below).

Causes

1. *Infective*
   - Hepatitis A, B, C.   ⎫ the commonest causes
   - Hepatitis non-A, B, C, D, E. ⎭ worldwide
   - Leptospirosis.
   - Yellow fever.
   - Sepsis.

2. *Drugs*
   - Hepatotoxic effect, e.g. paracetamol poisoning (the commonest cause in the UK).
   - Idiosyncratic drug reaction, e.g. halothane, non-steroidal anti-inflammatory drugs (NSAIDs), rifampicin, isoniazid, chloroquine, lamotrigine, 'Ecstacy'.

3. *Toxins*
   - Alcohol.
   - Mushroom (*Aminita phalloides*) poisoning.
   - Carbon tetrachloride and other industrial chemicals.

4. *Ischaemic*
   - Ischaemic hepatitis.
   - Acute Budd–Chiari syndrome.

5. *Metabolic*
   - Wilson's disease.
   - Fatty liver of pregnancy.
   - Reye's syndrome.

6. *Miscellaneous*
   - Massive malignant/lymphomatous infiltration.
   - Paraneoplastic phenomenon in lymphoma.

Clinical picture

Acute liver disease is categorized according to the speed of onset.

1. *Hyperacute liver failure (65–70% of cases).* Encephalopathy develops within 7 days of the onset of jaundice. Although cerebral oedema is most common in this group, and the prothrombin time (PT) is markedly prolonged, the prognosis is better than for the other groups.

2. *Acute liver failure (30% of cases).* Encephalopathy develops 8–28 days after the onset of jaundice. Such patients have a high incidence of cerebral oedema, severe prolongation of the PT and a high mortality.

3. Subacute liver failure (<5% of cases). Encephalopathy develops 4–12 weeks after the onset of jaundice. The mortality is higher than the other groups, despite a low incidence of cerebral oedema and a less marked prolongation of the PT.

Patients are typically well before the onset of symptoms, and have no past record of chronic liver disease. Nausea and malaise occur initially, followed by jaundice then encephalopathy. In some cases of hyperacute liver failure, the onset of encephalopathy may precede the jaundice. A general fruity odour (foetor hepaticus) is usually evident when encephalopathy ensues. Other common findings are constructional apraxia (as displayed by an inability to reproduce simple symbols) and a flapping tremor (asterixis).

Signs of chronic liver disease are usually absent. The liver and spleen are usually small (both are usually enlarged in acute-on-chronic liver failure). Progressive shrinkage of the liver in subacute cases is a bad prognostic sign.

Grades of hepatic encephalopathy are described in *Table 1*.

Table 1. Grades of hepatic encephalopathy

Grade	Description
I	Confusion or altered mood
II	Inappropriate behaviour ± increasing drowsiness
III	Stuporous but arousable, markedly confused, obeys only simple commands
IV	Coma with no response to painful stimuli

Investigations

Initial blood tests should include: full blood count, clotting screen, blood group and save, electrolytes, glucose, liver enzymes, hepatitis A, B, C serology (plus delta agent serology in hepatitis B cases), paracetamol level, serum copper and caeruloplasmin level (in those <50 years old), and arterial blood gas analysis. Blood specimens should also be taken for other causes of pre-existing and unrecognized liver injury (e.g. autoantibodies, ferritin), and some serum stored for later analysis (e.g. for toxin or drug levels, bacterial or viral antibodies). Blood cultures and urine, sputum, stool and ascites specimens should be obtained for microbiological analysis (even if there are no signs of infection). Invasive catheters should be replaced every 3–5 days. An electrocardiogram (ECG) and chest radiograph should be requested. An ultrasound scan of the liver, spleen and pancreas with Doppler studies of the hepatic and portal veins should be obtained.

Management

In all cases, close liaison with a specialist centre is crucial. Patients should initially be managed on an intensive therapy unit and transferred to a specialist referral unit after discussion. Indications for referral of patients with non-paracetamol- and paracetamol-induced liver failure are given in *Tables 2* and *3*.

Table 2. Indications for referral of patients to a specialist centre with non-paracetamol-induced acute liver failure

Hyperacute	Acute	Subacute
Encephalopathy	Encephalopathy	Encephalopathy
PT >30 s	PT >30 s	PT >20 s
Renal failure	Renal failure	Renal failure
		Serum Na <130 μmol/l

Table 3. Indications for referral to a specialist centre following paracetamol-induced acute liver failure

Day 2	Day 3	Day 4
Arterial pH <7.30[*]	Arterial pH <7.30[*]	INR >6.0 or
INR >3.0 or	INR >4.5 or	PT >75 s
PT >50 s	PT >60 s	Progressive rise
Oliguria	Oliguria	in PT
Creatinine	Creatinine	Oliguria
>200 μmol/l	>200 μmol/l	Creatinine
Hypoglycaemia	Encephalopathy	>300 μmol/l
		Encephalopathy

[*]With improved early management of paracetamol poisoning (i.e. liberal use of *N*-acetylcysteine and aggressive rehydration), acidosis in the absence of other prognostic signs should be interpreted with caution. Furthermore, the pH should only be assessed after reversible factors (e.g. shock, sepsis, effects of other drugs such as aspirin) have been corrected.

1. General measures

- The general principle of management is close invasive monitoring to allow the early detection and treatment of complications.
- A central venous pressure monitor, arterial line, urinary catheter and nasogastric tube should be inserted in all cases.
- If the grade of encephalopathy is III or IV, endotracheal intubation is necessary to prevent aspiration. Since the development of encephalopathy may be rapid, and since cerebral oedema is aggravated by any movement, endotracheal intubation should be considered at an early stage prior to transfer to a specialist unit.

- Mechanical ventilation is necessary for a partial pressure of oxygen (Po_2) <10 kPa or a partial pressure of carbon dioxide (Pco_2) >6.5 kPa.
- Human albumin solution (not saline) should be used to maintain the blood pressure; if this fails, inotropes should be used initially.
- When the peripheral vascular resistance falls, adrenaline and noradrenaline are used to increase the mean arterial pressure (recent evidence, however, suggests that these agents may aggravate tissue hypoxia). The circulatory vasodilators, prostacycline and N-acetylcysteine, may prevent such tissue hypoxia and are currently being evaluated.
- Blood sugar measurements are needed every 2–3 hours, as hypoglycaemia is a common problem. This should be prevented with a continuous infusion of 5% or 10% dextrose, and treated with an infusion of 50% dextrose.
- Renal failure develops in 75% of cases of ALF due to paracetamol overdose, and in 30% of other cases. This may be prevented with adequate fluid resuscitation. Low-dose dopamine may slow renal deterioration by improving renal blood flow, and haemoperfusion or haemodialysis is needed for established renal failure.
- Coagulopathy and haemorrhage are common. Prophylactic i.v. vitamin K is usually given but its benefit is unproved. Fresh frozen plasma and platelets are given to treat bleeding or to cover invasive procedures. A coagulopathy should only be corrected after discussion with the referral centre, as alteration of the INR will affect the timing of referral and transplantation.
- Upper gastrointestinal (GI) haemorrhage due to stress ulcers can be prevented with sucralfate (2 g three times daily).

2. Encephalopathy and cerebral oedema. Encephalopathy develops at some stage in all patients with ALF. The initial step in management is the prevention and treatment of any precipitating factors. These factors include hypoglycaemia, sepsis, hypoxia, gastrointestinal haemorrhage, electrolyte disturbance (commonly hypokalaemia), acid–base disturbance, drug toxicity (e.g. opiates, sedatives), alcohol withdrawal and constipation.

Treatment is with a protein-free diet, twice-daily phosphate enemas and lactulose via the nasogastric tube at a starting dose of 30 ml three times a day (aiming to achieve two to four loose stools a day). Flumazenil (a benzodiazepine-receptor antagonist) and metronidazole have also been used, but their role is uncertain. Neomycin is now seldom used, due to the risk of systemic absorption and nephrotoxicity.

Patients with grade III and grade IV encephalopathy have a high incidence of complications (i.e. cerebral oedema, occult seizures, ischaemic brain injury) which are the leading causes of death in this group. Early detection and treatment is critical to improve survival. Such patients should be nursed at a head tilt of 20–30° above the horizontal. Intracranial pressure (ICP) is monitored with an extradural pressure transducer in specialist units. The risks of insertion include intracranial haemorrhage and infection. Cerebral oedema occurs at a sustained ICP of >30 mmHg, and this should be treated with i.v. mannitol (1 g/kg bodyweight as an i.v. infusion of a 20% solution). An adequate renal output is essential to prevent fluid overload. Intravenous thiopentone and mechanical hyperventilation are used for those who do not respond to mannitol.

Seizures occur in 45% of patients. These are usually not clinically evident if the patient is sedated and ventilated, and all such patients should be investigated with an electro-encephalogram (EEG) to detect such occult seizures. As these aggravate cerebral oedema and ischaemia, patients with grade IV encephalopathy are treated with prophylactic phenytoin.

3. Infections. Bacterial infections complicate almost 90% and fungal infections about 30% of cases of ALF with grade II encephalopathy or more. Most infections are acquired within the first 3 days and are commonly respiratory infections. The characteristic signs of infection (e.g. leucocytosis and pyrexia) are usually absent. A systemic fungal infection should be suspected in those with established renal failure, a persistent leucocytosis or unexplained deterioration in the coma grade. Prophylactic parenteral antibiotics, with or without selective intestinal decontamination with enteral antibiotics, reduce the risk of sepsis. The specific regimen varies according to the types and sensitivities of bacteria found in each individual liver unit.

4. Bioartificial livers. Hepatic support systems or 'bioartificial livers' are devices aimed at supporting liver function until sufficient liver regeneration has taken place, or until a suitable donor liver is available. One such device, the extracorporeal liver assist device (ELAD), uses cultured human hepatoblastoma cells in the extracapillary space of a hollow fibre dialyzer, through which venous blood is pumped. Initial studies using this, and other similar devices, have shown favourable results, and such devices may eventually become a standard part of management of ALF.

5. Paracetamol-induced ALF. The mainstay of treatment is the use of *N*-acetylcysteine. This enhances glutathione levels, promotes the elimination of paracetamol metabolites and possibly enhances peripheral oxygen delivery. Initially this was only given within 16 hours of the overdose; however, evidence has shown an improvement when it is administered later than this.

Liver transplantation

The benefits of liver transplantation over intensive supportive therapy are greatest in those with subacute liver failure, as spontaneous recovery of liver function is much less likely than in the hyperacute group.

Liver transplantation should be considered in any patient with grade III or IV encephalopathy. The survival in such patients is less than 20%, but survival rates with transplantation are 60–80%. See also 'Transplantation – liver' (p. 254).

King's College criteria for liver transplantation in acute liver failure

1. *Paracetamol poisoning*
- pH <7.30 (see note above regarding pH as a referral criterion) *or*
- PT >100 s *and* serum creatinine >300 μmol/l *and* grade III or IV encephalopathy.

2. *Non-paracetamol cases*
- PT >100 s or INR >6.7 (irrespective of grade of encephalopathy) *or*
- Any three of the following (irrespective of grade of encephalopathy).
    Unfavourable aetiology (seronegative hepatitis, halothane hepatitis or drug reaction).
    Age <10 or >40 years.
    INR >4.0 or PT >50 s.
    Jaundice >7 days prior to encephalopathy.
    Serum bilirubin >300 μmol/l.

Further reading

Caraceni P, Van Thiel DH. Acute liver failure. *Lancet*, 1995; **345:** 163–9.
O'Grady J. Acute liver failure. *Journal of the Royal College of Physicians of London*, 1997; **31:** 603–7.
O'Grady JG, Alexander GJM, Hayllar KM, Williams R. Early indicators of prognosis in fulminant hepatic failure. *Gastroenterology*, 1989; **97:** 439–45.
Vale JA, Proudfoot AT. Paracetamol poisoning. *Lancet*, 1995; **346:** 547–52.
Williams R. New directions in acute liver failure. *Journal of the Royal College of Physicians of London*, 1994; **28:** 552–9.

Related topic of interest

Transplantation – liver (p. 254)

ASCITES

Ascites is the pathological accumulation of free fluid in the peritoneal cavity. Cirrhosis (usually due to alcoholic liver disease) accounts for over 80% of cases. Other causes include:

- Peritoneal carcinomatosis (10% of cases).
- Congestive cardiac failure.
- Nephrotic syndrome.
- Abdominal tuberculosis.
- Hepatic venous obstruction (e.g. Budd–Chiari syndrome).
- Portal vein thrombosis.
- Constrictive pericarditis.
- Meig's syndrome.
- Peritoneal mesothelioma.
- Chylous ascites (caused by lymphatic obstruction due to lymphoma, inadvertent surgical transection during laparotomy or intestinal lymphangiectasia).
- Myxoedema.
- Renal dialysis.
- Acute pancreatitis.

In chronic liver disease, it is proposed that a reduced intravascular volume (secondary to peripheral and splanchnic vasodilatation, hypoalbuminaemia and arteriovenous shunting) results in renal sodium and water retention via the renin–angiotensin system. This causes plasma volume expansion and portal hypertension, with a consequent overflow of fluid into the extravascular space. The increase in intrasinusoidal pressure in cirrhosis stimulates hepatic lymph formation which adds to the ascites.

Clinical features

In cirrhosis, ascites usually develops insidiously but may occur rapidly in the setting of an acute decompensation (e.g. due to variceal haemorrhage, infection, alcoholic binge, portal or splenic vein thrombosis, development of a hepatoma and hepatotoxic drugs). Rapidly developing ascites is also characteristically found in the Budd–Chiari syndrome and in some cases of peritoneal carcinomatosis.

Positional dullness on percussion of the flanks is detected when at least 2 l of fluid is present. A fluid thrill is detected when >4 l of ascitic fluid has accumulated.

Investigations

A diagnostic abdominal paracentesis (of about 50 ml) should be performed initially. It is safe and may be performed in the setting of a coagulopathy, but should be avoided in the presence of disseminated intravascular coagulation (DIC). Important features are:

1. *Colour*
- Straw-coloured fluid is seen in uncomplicated cirrhosis (may be bile-stained), nephrotic syndrome and cardiac failure.

- Blood-stained fluid is seen in carcinomatosis, haemorrhagic pancreatitis, or recent paracentesis or liver biopsy.
- Turbid fluid is seen in infections (including tuberculosis) and pancreatitis.
- Milky fluid occurs in chylous ascites (a triglyceride level of >5 mmol/l is suggestive and distinguishes it from pseudochylous ascites, which is caused by infection or malignancy and has a normal triglyceride content).

2. *Cell count*
- An absolute neutrophil count of >250 cells/ml is an indicator of spontaneous bacterial peritonitis.
- Lymphocytosis may be seen in peritoneal tuberculosis.

3. *Protein concentration.* Levels above the normal of 10–20 g/l may be found in those with Budd–Chiari syndrome, secondary bacterial peritonitis and in pancreatic ascites. A division of causes of ascites into 'exudate' and 'transudate' by means of the protein concentration is not as accurate as was previously thought, and has largely been superseded by the serum-ascites albumin gradient.

4. *Serum-ascites albumin gradient.* This is calculated by subtracting the ascites albumin concentration from the serum albumin concentration. A level of >1.1 g/dl indicates portal hypertension, and a gradient of <1.1 g/dl excludes it.

5. *Amylase concentration.* This is elevated in pancreatic ascites, but also in other causes of acute intra-abdominal pathology (e.g. bowel perforation).

6. *Microbiological assessment.* The conventional method is a Gram stain and culture of a centrifuged specimen; however, sensitivity is increased by directly innoculating blood-culture bottles with the ascitic aspirate. A Ziehl–Neilsen stain and suitable cultures are performed if tuberculosis is suspected.

7. *Cytology.* Although malignant cells may help to confirm a diagnosis of carcinomatosis, this is neither sensitive nor specific (normal peritoneal endothelial cells may resemble malignant cells).

Treatment of cirrhotic ascites

1. *Out-patient treatment.* Those with mild ascites may be managed as out-patients. A combination of spironolactone and frusemide (starting at 100 mg and 40 mg, respectively, taken together as single doses in the morning) is better than either alone. Amiloride has a quicker onset of action than spironolactone and may be used in place of spironolactone if side-effects (particularly painful gynaecomastia) occur. Patients should receive dietary advice to restrict salt intake to 60 mmol of sodium/day.

2. In-patient treatment. Indications for in-patient treatment are tense ascites, failure of weight loss of 2–4 kg/week, and complications of treatment (e.g. renal impairment, encephalopathy, electrolyte disturbance).

Treatment is often more practical and effective as an in-patient. This allows more careful monitoring of the response to treatment and complications (e.g. renal failure, spontaneous bacterial peritonitis), patient education and alcohol detoxification if required.

Diuretic therapy, as for out-patients, should be given. Doses should be sequentially increased according to the response – up to a maximal daily dose of 160 mg of frusemide and 400 mg of spironolactone. NSAIDs and i.v. diuretics (which may precipitate prerenal failure) should be avoided in those with ascites.

General measures include alternate-day weight measurements, strict fluid-balance monitoring and a salt-restricted diet of 60 mmol/day. Strict bed rest and fluid restriction have been advocated in the past, but are now thought not to be helpful.

Serum electrolytes should be measured three times weekly. A negative sodium balance is essential and the optimal dose of diuretics may be tailored to achieve this. The sodium balance is estimated by subtracting the 24-hour urine sodium excretion (daily urine volume multiplied by a random urine sodium concentration) from the daily sodium intake. A negative sodium balance and weight loss of 0.5 kg/day should be aimed for.

Those with tense ascites and those in whom medical treatment has failed (about 10% of patients) should have a therapeutic paracentesis of 4–6 l/day. Contraindications are those with Child's grade C and renal failure. Hypovolaemia and the hepatorenal syndrome are the principal adverse effects and can be prevented by the administration of 6 g of salt-free albumin per litre of ascites removed. Cheaper alternatives which seem to be as effective are Haemaccel (or other colloid solutions) or 5% human albumin solution (HAS). A single, total paracentesis is now also considered an option (i.e. about 10 l of ascites drained in 1 hour with 6 g i.v. salt-free albumin per litre drained). This has been shown to be safe and reduces in-hospital stay.

3. Refractory ascites. Those patients who fail to respond adequately to diuretics and paracentesis, or who develop complications of diuretic treatment, are offered a number of options:

- Ultrafiltration of the ascites with re-infusion of the concentrate using a peritoneal dialysis catheter and ultrafiltration apparatus is possible but carries a risk of sepsis.

- Radiologically placed transjugular intrahepatic portosystemic stent shunts (TIPSS) are used in some centres to treat refractory ascites. Recent evidence, however, has shown an unacceptably high incidence of complications (mainly encephalopathy and renal failure).
- A surgically placed peritoneo–venous (Le Veen) shunt from the peritoneal cavity to the superior vena cava is an option in selected patients. The complications of shunt malfunction (shunt occlusion occurs in 50%), infection, DIC and pulmonary oedema preclude their more widespread use.
- Refractory ascites is an accepted indication for liver transplantation in suitable patients. This is the only treatment for refractory ascites that improves survival.
- Those patients with malignant ascites respond better to repeated paracentesis than to diuretics and salt restriction. A peritoneo–venous shunt may provide relief for several months before it blocks.

Prognosis

The advent of ascites in most conditions implies a poor prognosis. In patients with cirrhosis, it carries a 50% 2-year survival. In carcinomatosis, patients have a mean survival of 20 weeks.

Spontaneous bacterial peritonitis

Spontaneous bacterial peritonitis (SBP) occurs in 20% of cirrhotic patients. The risk increases with the severity of the liver disease, and in those with a low ascites protein (<1 g/dl). Infection is usually due to a single Gram-negative organism of gut origin (cf. secondary bacterial peritonitis which is usually polymicrobial). Bacteraemia in such patients may follow a gastrointestinal haemorrhage and is augmented by increased gut permeability to bacteria, reduced serum complement levels and neutrophil functional impairment. Ascitic fluid, which is deficient in bacterial opsonins, provides a medium for bacterial growth.

Clinical signs are often absent and the condition should always be suspected if a patient with ascites deteriorates. An ascitic neutrophil count of >250 cells/ml is diagnostic. Ascitic fluid culture is often negative, as the bacterial count is usually low.

Most uncomplicated cases respond well to an oral quinolone (e.g. ciprofloxacin). Those with advanced liver disease require an i.v. third-generation cephalosporin.

Out-patient secondary (and possibly primary) prophylaxis with an oral quinolone or trimethoprim–sulphamethoxazole should be considered.

Of in-patients with SBP, 40–60% will die during that hospital admission, usually due to other concomitant factors. Seventy percent of cases recur within 1 year. Recurrent SBP is an indication for liver transplantation.

Further reading

Jalan R, Hayes PC. Hepatic encephalopathy and ascites. *Lancet*, 1997; **350:** 1309–15.
Runyon BA. Care of patients with ascites. *New England Journal of Medicine*, 1994; **330(5):** 337–42.

Related topics of interest

Cirrhosis (p. 40)
Portal hypertension (p. 223)

AUTOIMMUNE CHRONIC HEPATITIS

Chronic hepatitis is defined as a chronic inflammation of the liver continuing without improvement for at least 6 months. Autoimmune chronic hepatitis is characterized, in addition, by the presence of 'piecemeal necrosis' (a term now becoming outdated, the equivalent in newer staging systems being 'periportal hepatitis'), hypergammaglobulinaemia, and elevated levels of circulating liver-associated autoantibodies (see below). These autoantibodies are important diagnostically, but their role in the pathogenesis and course of the disease is unknown. Other causes of chronic hepatitis include chronic viral hepatitis, haemochromatosis, drugs, Wilson's disease and α_1-antitrypsin deficiency, and are discussed elsewhere.

Classification of autoimmune chronic hepatitis

The condition is classified according to the pattern of circulating autoantibodies.

1. *Type I autoimmune chronic hepatitis.* This is typified by a variable pattern of autoantibodies, including combinations of antinuclear, double-stranded DNA and smooth muscle (actin) antibodies.

2. *Type II autoimmune chronic hepatitis.* This is characterized by the presence of autoantibodies against liver and kidney microsomes (LKM) type I. This is further subdivided into type IIa (autoimmune) and type IIb (hepatitis C-related). The distinction between types IIa and IIb is important, as type IIa responds to corticosteroids while type IIb may require interferon treatment (which can exacerbate autoimmune hepatitis).

3. *Chronic hepatitis D.* This is characterized by the presence of LKM type III autoantibodies (found in some patients with chronic delta virus infection).

4. *Primary biliary cirrhosis (PBC)/autoimmune cholangiopathy.* These diseases, characterized by cholestasis, differ from the other subgroups of autoimmune chronic liver disease in that disease activity is centred on the intrahepatic bile ducts rather than on the hepatocyte. PBC is characterized by the presence of anti-mitochondrial antibodies (AMAs) and is covered elsewhere. The histological changes of immune cholangiopathy are identical to those of PBC, but AMAs are characteristically absent and anti-DNA and anti-smooth muscle (actin) antibodies are present. As immune cholangiopathy tends to respond to steroids, it is thought to be an overlap between PBC and autoimmune chronic hepatitis.

Type I autoimmune hepatitis serves as the paradigm for investigation and treatment of autoimmune liver disease. Primary biliary cirrhosis and liver autoimmune phenomena associated with hepatitis C infection require a different approach and are discussed elsewhere.

Chronic autoimmune hepatitis (CAH) (type I)

This is the prototype of autoimmune hepatitis. It was formerly known as 'lupoid hepatitis' on account of a positive LE test being found in a significant proportion. This is a misleading term, as classical systemic lupus erythematosus (SLE) rarely involves the liver, and the characteristic autoantibodies found in CAH are not found in SLE. CAH is caused by a defect in suppressor T lymphocytes, which leads to the production of autoantibodies against hepatocyte surface antigens.

1. Clinical features. The disease mainly affects women between the ages of 15 and 30 or at the menopause, but can present at any age. The onset may be insidious, with fatigue a prominent early feature, or acute, and may initially be mistaken for a viral hepatitis. Nausea and amenorrhoea are common. In about 25% of cases, patients remain well, and the diagnosis is made after chronic liver disease/cirrhosis is established.

Associated autoimmune diseases include insulin-dependent diabetes, ulcerative colitis, pulmonary infiltrates, Hashimoto's thyroiditis, non-deforming polyarthritis, lymphadenopathy, hypersplenism and renal tubular defects.

Clinical signs are often episodic and come and go with changes in disease activity. These include jaundice (often fluctuating), spider naevi, cushingoid features (striae, acne, hirsutism, bruising) and hepatosplenomegaly.

2. Investigations. Transaminases are usually markedly elevated but fall with treatment and with disease progression. Bilirubin is variably elevated.

Protein electrophoresis shows a polyclonal gammopathy and immunoglobulin G (IgG) is almost always raised – the diagnosis is in doubt if it is not. Serum alpha-fetoprotein is often raised but falls with treatment. A mild normochromic normocytic anaemia, leucopenia and thrombocytopenia are common, and are often found before portal hypertension and hypersplenism occurs. Signs of chronic liver disease (coagulopathy and reduced albumin) occur in advanced cases.

Various autoantibodies are found, the diagnostically important ones being antinuclear antibody (present in 80% of patients), double-stranded DNA antibody and smooth muscle (actin) antibody. Titres of >1:40 are significant (>1:80 by some guidelines) and are found in 70% of patients. Lower titres occur in PBC and acute hepatitis A and B infection.

A liver biopsy is important to assess the stage of the disease and the response to treatment. Histological changes are those of chronic hepatitis and include lymphocyte and plasma cell infiltrates in the portal and periportal areas. With ongoing disease, periportal hepatitis (piecemeal necrosis) and bridging fibrosis occur; cirrhosis usually develops 2 years after the onset in untreated cases.

3. Differential diagnosis
- Chronic viral hepatitis.
- Sclerosing cholangitis should be excluded with an endoscopic retrograde cholangiopancreatography (ERCP) if the alkaline phosphatase is disproportionally elevated or if ulcerative colitis coexists.
- Wilson's disease is a rare but important differential diagnosis; it is diagnosed by slit-lamp examination of the cornea, serum caeruloplasmin, and serum and liver copper levels.
- Haemochromatosis should be excluded with serum iron studies and liver iron staining.
- Drug-induced chronic hepatitis.
- Chronic alcoholic liver disease.

4. Treatment. Prednisolone (30 mg/day for 1 week, then a maintenance dose of 10–15 mg/day for 6 months) produces a rapid clinical and biochemical improvement in most cases. The rapidity of the response to steroids is almost diagnostic of CAH. At 6 months, if a biochemical and histological remission has occurred, the steroids should be gradually withdrawn. Relapses are unfortunately common and most patients require long-term/life-long steroids.

Azathioprine (50–100 mg/day) is used for cases resistant to steroids or for those with unacceptable steroid-induced side-effects (which occurs with doses of >15 mg/day).

Liver transplantation may be necessary if steroids fail to induce a remission or if complications of cirrhosis develop. The disease does not recur in the transplanted liver.

5. Prognosis. The clinical course is extremely variable, and is punctuated by episodes of relapses when malaise and jaundice are pronounced. Overall, corticosteroids prolong life, but those who fail to respond will eventually develop cirrhosis and its complications. In such patients, bleeding from oesophageal varices and hepatocellular failure are the usual causes of death. The 10-year survival is 65% and the mean survival is 12 years (a wide range is reported in the literature).

Further reading

Meyer zum Buschenfelde K-H, Lohse AW. Autoimmune hepatitis. *New England Journal of Medicine*, 1995; **333:** 1004.

Related topics of interest

BARRETT'S OESOPHAGUS

The oesophagus is normally lined with stratified squamous epithelium, and there is usually an easily visible, sharp transition to columnar-lined epithelium (the 'Z' line) at the junction with the stomach. In some patients (usually those with gastro-oesophageal reflux disease (GORD)), the mucosa of the distal tubular oesophagus undergoes metaplastic change to columnar-type (with or without intestinal metaplasia), and when 3 cm or more of the distal oesophagus is affected the condition can be labelled 'Barrett's oesophagus'. The diagnosis can still be made when a shorter segment of the oesophagus is affected if intestinal metaplasia is present. The exact extent is often difficult to measure, and may be diffuse, circular or non-circular in type, or it may occur as isolated islands.

The exact cause is uncertain, but it is proposed that the metaplastic change is a defence reaction of the oesophagus in response to excessive acid exposure in the long term. Barrett's oesophagus is common and occurs in about 10–20% of those who present with GORD.

The propensity for a columnar-lined oesophagus to develop an adenocarcinoma is the main reason for interest in this condition. The risk is difficult to determine but it is estimated as 30–40 times greater than in the general population, and the annual incidence in those with endoscopically obvious disease is 0.8%. Approximately 32% of those with dysplasia will develop adenocarcinoma. The risk is greater in those with long-segment disease; the significance of short-segment columnar-lined epithelium remains controversial.

Clinical features

Over 90% of those with Barrett's oesophagus are asymptomatic, and any symptoms that do develop are due to GORD or its complications. Dysphagia (with or without a stricture) is a relatively common presentation in those that are symptomatic.

Although Barrett's oesophagus is technically a histological diagnosis, the different macroscopic appearance of columnar and squamous epithelia suggests the diagnosis at endoscopy. Endoscopic detection requires skill, and it is estimated that at least 10% of cases are missed at endoscopy. Barrett's mucosa is often congested: 10–20% have evidence of oesophagitis with erythema, friability, linear erosions or ulcers, and necrotic pseudomembranes.

Management

Management and surveillance of Barrett's oesophagus is controversial. It is very difficult to identify high-risk individuals due to the difficulty in staging biopsy specimens, and those carcinomas that are identified have often already metastasized. Regular endoscopic screening in Barrett's has not convincingly reduced the mortality from oesophageal cancer in studies to date. A suggested approach to management is as follows:

- If a columnar epithelium-lined distal oesophagus is recognized at endoscopy, four-quadrant biopsies should be taken.
- If histology confirms specialized epithelial columnar metaplasia, without dysplasia, the risk of adenocarcinoma is

increased and surveillance with endoscopy and biopsies should be considered – possibly every 1–2 years.

- If dysplasia is present on the initial biopsy, further multiple biopsies should be taken and if these show high-grade dysplasia, patients should be considered for oesophagectomy. If high-grade dysplasia is not detected, follow-up endoscopy may be considered every year, for as long as the patient is a candidate for oesophagectomy.
- All patients with Barrett's oesophagus should receive proton pump inhibitor treatment. This has been shown to provide variable symptomatic relief and may lead to a regression of the histological changes in some cases.
- Surgical antireflux procedures (e.g. Nissen's fundoplication) may be similarly effective in those with, and without, complications of reflux.

Other treatment strategies

Therapies aimed at local ablation are promising, but concern has been raised at the possibility that such modalities may only destroy superficial dysplastic cells, leaving deeper, potentially malignant cells undetected.

Endoscopic ablation of the affected area with an argon laser, followed by long-term inhibition of acid secretion with a proton pump inhibitor, has been shown to lead to squamous epithelium regrowth. The treatment is, however, not widely available and is labour intensive.

Photodynamic therapy is a relatively new treatment currently being evaluated. The technique involves the oral administration of a photosensitizing substance (5-aminolaevulinic acid (protoporphyrin IX)) which binds to dysplastic cells in the gastrointestinal tract. Photodynamic therapy is then administered via an endoscopically positioned optical fibre. The cells bound to the 5-aminolaevulinic acid are preferentially destroyed. Initial results have been encouraging, but larger studies are needed to establish whether this treatment will prevent dysplasia and cancer in the long term.

Further reading

Barr H, Shephard NA, Dix A. Eradication of high-grade dysplasia in columnar-lined (Barrett's) oesophagus by photodynamic therapy with endogenously generated protoporphyrin IX. *Lancet*, 1996; **348**: 584–5.

Probert CSJ, Jayanthi V, Mayberry JF. Barrett's oesophagus – a review. *Quarterly Journal of Medicine*, 1991; **295**: 883–89.

Spechler SJ, Goyal RK. The columnar-lined esophagus, intestinal metaplasia, and Norman Barrett. *Gastroenterology*, 1996; **110**: 614–21.

Related topics of interest

BENIGN GASTRIC AND DUODENAL TUMOURS

Gastric leiomyoma

These are the commonest benign gastric tumours and arise from the smooth muscle layer. They are a common incidental finding at autopsies and are rarely symptomatic. Large lesions may ulcerate and present as upper gastrointestinal bleeding. At endoscopy they appear as intra-luminal polypoid lesions with overlying superficial ulceration. They may be removed by surgical excision. Exclusion of a leiomyosarcoma may be difficult. Endoscopic biopsies often fail to reach the level of the tumour; submucosal injection of saline enables a snare resection of the mucosa overlying such tumours, and subsequent, deeper, more diagnostic endoscopic biopsies. Endoscopic ultrasound may also be useful at excluding a malignant lesion.

Gastric polyps

Gastric polyps are uncommon epithelial lesions that are usually found incidentally on barium or endoscopic examination. They are either hyperplastic or adenomatous.

Hyperplastic (or regenerative) polyps	These account for about 90% of gastric polyps. They usually occur in the body and fundus, are usually small (<2 cm), smooth, often multiple and may be sessile or pedunculated. They are of no significance and do not undergo malignant change, but should be biopsied at endoscopy as they may mimic early cancer.
Adenomatous polyps	Adenomatous polyps are far rarer tubulovillous structures that occur mainly in the antrum. They have the same malignant potential as colonic adenomatous polyps and should be removed endoscopically. They occasionally bleed when ulcerated and, if large, may prolapse through the pylorus causing an outlet obstruction. They may be associated with colonic adenomatous polyps, which should be excluded by colonoscopy.
Associations	• Achlorhydria is a common coincidental finding with hyperplastic gastric polyps, and an association with pernicious anaemia and gastric carcinoma is well described. • An increased incidence of gastric polyps and gastric carcinoma is found in Gardener's syndrome and, less commonly, the Peutz–Jegher's syndrome. • Fundal and antral polyps occur in the familial adenomatous polyposis: a small, but significant, increased risk of gastric carcinoma is recognized.

Benign tumours of the duodenum

Benign tumours of the duodenum are rare, the most common being tubular adenomas. The latter usually occur in the first part of the duodenum and may present with gastrointestinal bleeding. The duodenum is the most common upper gastrointestinal site for adenomatous polyps in familial polyposis coli, and malignant transformation in this site does occasionally occur. Adenomas with villous or tubulovillous histology are more rare, representing approximately 1% of duodenal tumours. They tend to be peri-ampullary, and sometimes grow to obstruct the duodenum or ampulla. They have a greater tendency to bleed and undergo malignant transformation (up to two-thirds have malignant or premalignant change in some series). They are often associated with a more generalized intestinal polyposis syndrome, especially when multiple.

Further reading

Bush JL, Pantongrag-Brown L. Gastritides, gastropathies and polyps unique to the stomach. *Radiologic Clinics of North America*, 1994; **32(6):** 1215–31.

Morgan BK, Compton C, Talbert M, Gallagher WJ, Wood WC. Benign smooth muscle tumours of the gastrointestinal tract. A 24-year experience. *Annals of Surgery*, 1990; **211(1):** 63–6.

Related topic of interest

Hereditary neoplastic syndromes of the intestine (p. 166)

CARCINOMA OF THE PANCREAS

The incidence of pancreatic carcinoma has tripled over the past 40 years throughout the western world. It occurs most commonly in men over the age of 60. It has one of the lowest survival rates of all cancers (1–2% at 5 years), and the mean survival at the time of diagnosis is <6 months. Symptoms are often vague and non-specific in the early stages and no diagnostic tests exist which are able to detect early (potentially curable) tumours.

Risk factors

- A western diet (high protein and high fat) has been implicated.
- Pancreatic cancer occurs at a younger age in cigarette smokers.
- Alcohol consumption (particularly beer) is weakly associated.
- Diabetes (particularly in women) carries an increased risk.
- Those with chronic pancreatitis have a slightly increased risk.
- Recurrent acute pancreatitis (an inherited disorder: referral of suspected families to a clinical geneticist is appropriate).

Clinical features

Non-specific constitutional symptoms are common in the early stages. Progressive weight loss and anorexia are frequently found. An alteration in bowel habit, lassitude and depression are relatively common.

A dull, vague epigastric pain is the presenting feature in 75% of cases. The pain may radiate to the back, implying invasion of retroperitoneal organs or splanchnic nerves. In the late stages, relief may be obtained by flexing the trunk forward.

Patients may occasionally present with the recent onset of brittle diabetes or diabetic ketoacidosis.

The tumour site determines some of the other presenting features.

1. Carcinomas in the head of the pancreas. 70% of pancreatic carcinomas occur in the head of the gland. The usual presentation is one of jaundice and epigastric pain. The tumour may occasionally compress the duodenum producing obstructive symptoms, or may invade the stomach producing haematemesis. Common bile-duct obstruction may cause cholangitis and recurrent attacks of acute pancreatitis may precede the diagnosis of pancreatic cancer.

2. Carcinomas of the body and tail. These tend to present later and have disseminated at the time of diagnosis. Jaundice is a late feature and may be due to hepatic metastasis. Predominant features are pain, anorexia and weight loss.

Physical signs

Most patients (90%) present with positive physical signs, suggesting incurability. An epigastric mass is found in a quarter of patients. Ascites is caused by local spread to the peritoneum or portal hypertension (due to compression or thrombosis of the splenic vein). A distended, palpable, non-tender gall bladder (Courvoisier's sign) may be found when a tumour in the head of the pancreas occludes the common bile duct.

Troissier's sign (a palpable left supraclavicular lymph node), Trousseau's sign (migratory thrombophlebitis) and metastatic fat necrosis (erythema nodosum-like lesions and polyarthritis) may be evident, but are not specific for pancreatic carcinoma.

Rarer features are abacterial endocarditis and Cushing's syndrome.

Differential diagnosis

Carcinoma of the head of the pancreas should always be differentiated from carcinomas of the ampulla or common bile duct which have a better prognosis. In the early stages, pancreatic cancer may closely mimic chronic pancreatitis.

Investigations

- The carcinoembryonic antigen (CEA) is elevated in over half of patients, but is neither specific nor sensitive. The newer tumour marker, CA 19-9, has been found in about 80% of cases – mostly in advanced disease. CA 19-9 is also elevated in acute and chronic pancreatitis and chronic liver disease. Tumour markers are most useful to monitor for recurrence after a potentially curative operation.
- Abdominal ultrasonography is the usual first-line imaging modality. An asymmetrically enlarged pancreatic mass with extra- and intrahepatic bile duct dilatation is the usual finding.
- Abdominal CT scan is valuable when poor views are obtained with ultrasonography. Percutaneous needle biopsy may be performed at the same time. The histology may be difficult to distinguish from chronic pancreatitis.
- If equivocal results are obtained with radiological and cytological tests, an ERCP is indicated. This has a sensitivity of >90% in diagnosing pancreatic cancer and is valuable in excluding other causes of a pancreatic mass or biliary obstruction (e.g. chronic pancreatitis, gallstones, ampullary tumours). Brushings for cytology may be performed, increasing the diagnostic accuracy.
- Laparotomy and diagnostic biopsy are occasionally needed in younger patients to distinguish a mass from chronic pancreatitis.
- Endoscopic ultrasound shows promise as a method to assess the extent of smaller lesions.

Treatment

1. *Surgery*
- Less than 10% of tumours are potentially curable. The curative operations most often performed are a pancreatico-

duodenectomy (Whipple's procedure) or a total pancreate-ctomy. Such operations should only be considered in fit, younger patients with tumours <3 cm and no evidence of local extension or metastasis.

- The overall surgical mortality is about 16%, but is sub-stantially lower in experienced hands.
- Five-year survival after a Whipple's operation is 4–15%.

2. *Palliative treatment.* Although most tumours are not curable, it is important to stress to patients that successful palliation is possible.

(a) Relief of jaundice (non-surgical)

- Endoscopic (ERCP) stent insertion is valuable in relieving malignant common bile-duct obstruction in most cases. This approach is preferable in the elderly as the morbidity, mortality and hospital stay are significantly less than with surgery.
- Percutaneous transhepatic cholangiography (PTC) is usu-ally used when ERCP has failed. It is useful to confirm the diagnosis and enables the placement of a percutaneous stent as definitive therapy.
- In the small number of cases not managed by the above, a combined percutaneous and endoscopic approach allows successful stenting in over 90%.

(b) Relief of jaundice (surgery)

- A cholecystojejunostomy with diverting enterostomy may be performed to decompress the biliary tree in those patients with jaundice and pruritus, although this is rarely used due to the widespread availability of ERCP nowa-days.
- A gastrojejunostomy is indicated to bypass a duodenal obstruction from an infiltrating tumour.

(c) Relief of pain

- Opiates (e.g. morphine sulphate, continuous 20 mg twice daily) are recommended as first-line analgesics and, if needed, should be introduced as soon as the diagnosis is made. Patient-controlled analgesia (PCA) devices may be needed.
- External beam radiotherapy is useful at relieving intractable pain but does not alter survival.
- A percutaneous coeliac plexus block may provide life-long relief in those with a short life expectancy.

3. *Chemotherapy.* The role of chemotherapy with or with-out radiotherapy in carcinoma of the pancreas is unclear. The results of ongoing trials with several agents, including a met-alloproteinase inhibitor, are awaited. Patients undergoing such

treatments at present should do so in the context of clinical trials.

Carcinoma of the ampulla

These tumours are rare (10 times less common than pancreatic carcinoma) and occur twice as commonly in males. They arise from either the lower common bile duct, the head of the pancreas, the duodenum or the ampulla itself. They are adenocarcinomas, but have no unique histological features. Because they tend to present early, they have the best prognosis of all pancreaticobiliary tumours following resection. It is therefore important to distinguish them from pancreatic carcinomas.

Clinical presentation
- Most present with jaundice which, unlike more proximal tumours, may be intermittent. Unlike in pancreatic cancer, the jaundice is usually painless.
- Other features include cholangitis, acute pancreatitis and occult or overt intestinal bleeding if erosion into the duodenum occurs.

Investigations
- Abdominal ultrasound usually shows a dilated biliary tree with a distal obstruction.
- The diagnosis is usually made on ERCP which may display the 'double duct' sign (a dilated common bile duct and pancreatic duct). Biopsy, brushings for cytology and stent insertion may be performed at the same time.

Treatment
- Surgical resection is possible in 75% of cases, and the Whipple procedure is the operation of choice. Five-year survival rates of 40% have been achieved with this procedure.
- Palliation of irresectable tumours with a stent has been associated with prolonged survival rates, reflecting the slow growth of these tumours.

Further reading

Moossa AR, Stabile BE. The pancreas. In: Cuschieri A, Giles GR, Moossa AR (eds). *Essential Surgical Practice*, 3rd edn. Oxford: Butterworth-Heinemann, 1995; 1238–77.

Related topics of interest

CHOLANGIOCARCINOMA

Cholangiocarcinomas may arise from any portion of the biliary tree and their site determines the mode of presentation. All are adenocarcinomas and most present over the age of 65.

Carcinoma of the gall bladder

Although these tumours are slightly more common than cholangiocarcinomas elsewhere, they account for only 3–4% of all tumours of the gastrointestinal tract. Seventy percent of patients have coexistent gallstones. Congenital anomalies of the junction between the pancreatic duct and the common bile duct confer an increased risk.

Most patients (80%) present with advanced local disease and jaundice due to obstruction of extrahepatic bile ducts by a tumour or by regional lymph nodes. A significant proportion present with acute cholecystitis or empyema of the gall bladder and the diagnosis may be missed at operation if the gall bladder is not routinely examined histologically. Most will have metastatic spread by the time of presentation, although this may often not be evident on standard imaging. Localized tumours may be discovered incidentally at operation for gall bladder stones.

Carcinoma of the bile duct

Although any portion of the biliary tract may be involved, most of these occur at the hilum (Klatskin tumours). An increased incidence is found in association with choledochal cysts and anomalies of the junction between the common bile duct and the pancreatic duct. A strong association exists with primary sclerosing cholangitis (thought by some to be a premalignant condition) and therefore also with ulcerative colitis. The rapid worsening of jaundice in such patients should always provoke a search for an underlying cholangiocarcinoma.

Due to the eccentric position of most tumours, by the time painless obstructive jaundice and pruritus develop the disease is usually advanced with lymph node and visceral metastasis (80% of cases). The level of jaundice may fluctuate, which may mislead clinicians into favouring a benign process.

Other symptoms include episodic, ill-defined epigastric pain, fever (due to cholangitis), steatorrhoea and weight loss.

Carcinoma of the ampulla

This is discussed in the topic 'Carcinoma of the pancreas' (p. 27).

Investigations	An isolated elevated ALP may be an early sign of biliary disease without obstruction before the onset of clinical jaundice. In most cases, the blood tests show a cholestatic picture. An elevated CEA is found in some patients. Anaemia is usually due to chronic intestinal blood loss, sometimes exacerbated by a bleeding diathesis from chronic cholestasis. Many patients

are nutritionally depleted at presentation, conferring a high operative risk and poor overall survival.

A plain abdominal radiograph may show calcified gallstones and a calcified gall bladder wall ('porcelain gall bladder') indicative of chronic cholecystitis which is a premalignant lesion.

If good views are obtained, ultrasonography will show the level of obstruction and the presence of lesions in the gall bladder and common bile ducts in most cases. The presence of hilar nodes and hepatic secondaries or abscesses may also be detected.

When the diagnosis is suspected on clinical and radiological grounds, an ERCP is the diagnostic and therapeutic investigation of first choice. The cholangiogram obtained usually shows an abrupt cut-off, usually at the hilum. Ampullary tumours can be biopsied, and brushings or aspiration of more proximal lesions enable cytological confirmation.

A CT or magnetic resonance imaging (MRI) scan provides further anatomical detail of the tumour and is useful at detecting local and distant spread. An ultrasound- or CT-guided percutaneous biopsy may be possible.

PTC may be used alone or combined with an ERCP when cannulation of the ampulla is not possible, or for more proximal lesions.

Differential diagnosis

Benign strictures and localized strictures of primary sclerosing cholangitis (PSC) often closely mimic cholangiocarcinoma, both radiologically and histologically. Even postoperative specimens are often difficult to interpret due to the high grade of differentiation of most cholangiocarcinomas.

Treatment

1. *Non-surgical.* Most tumours are inoperable at presentation and a stent is inserted at the time of ERCP or PTC. Stents may be placed as a temporary procedure to relieve jaundice in potentially operable cases, but discuss with the regional referral centre first, as surgeons differ in their views over this practice. Traditionally, plastic stents have been used, but the newer (and more expensive) self-expanding metal stents may have a superior patency rate and have a lower incidence of cholangitis.

External beam or intraluminal radiotherapy is used in some centres as palliation in inoperable cases, or as adjunctive therapy after resection. The use of chemotherapy is contentious.

2. *Surgical.* There are no definite criteria regarding eligibility for surgery. In general, those patients with tumours found incidentally or young patients with localized, distal tumours are most suitable. Surgery may either involve a palliative

biliary-enteric bypass procedure or resection with partial hepa-tectomy. Liver transplantation has been performed, although results have been disappointing. Recent innovations in surgical techniques have rekindled an interest in transplantation surgery (the results of which up to now have been disappointing). Dis-cussion with a specialist centre is therefore advisable.

Prognosis   Carcinoma of the gall bladder has a 5-year survival of less than 5%. Overall survival for all types of cholangiocarcinomas is between 9 months and 3 years (mean of 1 year).

Further reading

Vauthey J-N, Blumgart LH. Recent advances in the management of cholangiocarcinomas. *Seminars in Liver Disease*, 1994; **14**: 109.

Related topics of interest

Ulcerative colitis – background and clinical features (p. 265)
Ulcerative colitis – medical and surgical management (p. 269)

CHRONIC PANCREATITIS

Chronic pancreatitis is a chronic inflammatory process leading to the destruction of exocrine tissue, fibrosis and, in some cases, the loss of endocrine function.

Causes

- Approximately 70% of adult patients with chronic pancreatitis are chronic alcohol abusers. A high-protein diet seems to potentiate the deleterious effects of alcohol.
- Other causes include obstruction of the pancreatic duct (e.g. post-traumatic ductal strictures, pseudocysts, peri-ampullary tumours), α_1-antitrypsin deficiency and pancreas divisum.
- It occasionally complicates cystic fibrosis, hyperparathyroidism and, very rarely, gallstones.
- An inherited (autosomal dominant) form has been described.
- Tropical pancreatitis is a poorly understood entity that occurs in impoverished areas in Africa and Asia, and is possibly caused by the ingestion of toxic substances or protein malnutrition.
- In a large proportion of cases, no obvious cause can be found.

Clinical features

1. History. In many patients, particularly in the early stages, chronic pancreatitis is clinically silent. After a time, most patients experience abdominal pain, and eventually exocrine then endocrine insufficiency (when approximately 90% of secretory function has been lost). The pain is usually upper abdominal and radiates to the back or scapula. It is often associated with nausea and vomiting. It is worse with eating or drinking and may be relieved with sitting forward or upright. Painful exacerbations occur on the background of chronic pain; however, they may subside with time as inflammation is gradually replaced by fibrosis. A pancreatic carcinoma should always be excluded when the pain becomes persistent or accelerated weight loss occurs.

Exocrine deficiency may cause malabsorption. Reduced excretion of lipase and bicarbonate cause fat malabsorption. This manifests as steatorrhoea which may be massive, but can be minimal if patients voluntarily reduce their fat intake. The stool volumes are often less than for those with intestinal mucosal disease. Malabsorption of fat-soluble vitamins rarely results in a clinical deficiency. Hypocalcaemia is usually due to unabsorbed intestinal fat chelating calcium and hence preventing its absorption. Protein and carbohydrate malabsorption occur less commonly.

Endocrine insufficiency occurs later and initially manifests as impaired glucose tolerance and eventually frank diabetes in 30% of patients.

Between 10 and 20% have painless pancreatitis and present with diabetes, jaundice or malabsorption.

2. Examination. Examination may show signs of malnutrition (due to malabsorption and food avoidance), upper abdominal tenderness and possibly an epigastric mass (suggestive of a pseudocyst or carcinoma).

Jaundice may be due to obstruction of the common bile duct as it passes through the pancreatic head (by inflammatory or neoplastic masses), or associated cirrhosis (present in approximately 10%).

Portal hypertension due to splenic or portal vein thrombosis may be found. It is important to distinguish it from alcoholic cirrhotic portal hypertension, because decompression procedures are a treatment option (see below).

Investigations

1. Laboratory tests. Serum amylase and lipase levels may be only slightly elevated in an acute attack, and are often normal in long-standing cases when fibrotic tissue has replaced much of the gland. In 5–10% of patients, bilirubin and alkaline phosphatase levels are elevated due to obstruction of the intra-pancreatic portion of the common bile duct. Associated alcoholic liver disease may produce deranged liver enzymes, hypoalbuminaemia and deranged clotting. An oral glucose tolerance test may show impaired glucose tolerance or diabetes. Malabsorption may produce hypoalbuminaemia, hypocalcaemia with an elevated alkaline phosphatase (vitamin D malabsorption) or deranged clotting (vitamin K malabsorption).

2. Imaging studies
- A plain abdominal radiograph will show ductal calcification in up to 30% of patients in the late stages.
- Ultrasonography may show pancreatic enlargement, tumours, ductal dilatation, or pseudocysts with an accuracy approaching that of a CT scan.
- A CT scan may show calcification or cystic areas not seen on ultrasonography.
- MRI and endoscopic ultrasound are further imaging modalities under evaluation at present.
- ERCP remains the gold standard for the diagnosis and planning of treatment of chronic pancreatitis. Characteristic features include multiple ductal strictures, intraductal calculi or small ducts with attenuated side branches (the 'tree in winter' appearance). In advanced cases, the main pancreatic duct may be dilated to 1 cm or more, producing a 'chain of lakes' appearance.

Functional assessment The following tests may be useful in the diagnosis of patients with recurrent pain and normal imaging investigations. In practice, however, an assessment of pancreatic exocrine function is rarely performed, especially when clinical features of malabsorption are present, because a positive result would not alter the management. Moreover, a normal test does not necessarily exclude chronic pancreatitis.

1. Direct pancreatic function tests. These tests remain the gold standard in assessing pancreatic exocrine insufficiency. However, they are impractical, uncomfortable for the patient and mainly only used as research tools. They involve intubation of the duodenum and measurement of the volume and bicarbonate and protein concentrations of pancreatic juice, after the ingestion of a standard Lundh test meal or the i.v. administration of secretin. The latter test may be helpful in identifying 'minimal change pancreatitis': this condition is described as alcohol-unrelated chronic pancreatitis with normal ERCP findings. The abnormality is thought to reside in the small pancreatic ducts.

2. Indirect tests
- Microscopic examination of a random faecal specimen for fat droplets offers a crude assessment of fat malabsorption from any cause (but will miss mild degrees of steatorrhoea).
- A faecal fat measurement, although unpopular with patients and staff, offers a quantitative assessment of steatorrhoea. Ideally, a standard diet including 70 g of fat per day should be taken for 6 days prior to, and during, the collection. Two sets of radio-opaque or isotope markers should be ingested 24 hours apart, and their presence noted in the stool to enable an accurate timing of collection. A faecal fat measurement of >5 g/day, or a level >5–8% of that ingested, is suggestive of fat malabsorption from a variety of causes.
- An oral radiolabelled triglyceride test is a more convenient method to assess fat malabsorption and is available in some centres.
- More convenient, but less sensitive, non-invasive tests for pancreatic exocrine insufficiency include the pancreolauryl and para-amino benzoic acid (PABA) tests (see 'Malabsorption' (p. 189)).
- Faecal elastase-1 measurement has recently been shown to be a sensitive, specific and convenient test of pancreatic insufficiency. A random faecal chymotrypsin level is also an option.

Management

1. *Pain control.* Pain is usually the most troublesome symptom. Abstinence from alcohol and avoidance of large meals is helpful in some cases. First-line medical therapy is with paracetamol, progressing to dihydrocodeine or NSAIDs. Opiates (pethidine) are often needed, but dependence is a common problem. Referral to a pain clinic is advisable.

Pain that persists despite maximal analgesic treatment should undergo an ERCP. Stones in the pancreatic duct can be removed and dilated ducts due to strictures can be decompressed by an endoscopically placed stent, or by surgery (e.g. pancreaticojejunostomy). The results, however, are often disappointing.

In those patients with non-dilated ducts and unremitting pain, a pancreaticoduodenectomy (Whipple's procedure) or partial pancreatectomy is occasionally considered.

Several studies have shown that pancreatic enzyme supplements (e.g. pancrelipase) and somatostatin analogues (e.g. octreotide) may be effective in relieving pain in the early stages. Their exact role has not, however, been firmly established.

A percutaneous coeliac plexus block may provide some relief but usually only for a few months. Surgical coeliac plexus excision is possible if recurrent percutaneous blocks are needed.

2. *Malabsorption.* Treatment consists of a low-fat diet and pancreatic enzyme supplements. Input from a dietician is valuable.

Steatorrhoea may be controlled by a daily fat intake of 20–50 g. Oral supplementation with medium-chain triglycerides (MCT) (e.g. trisorbon) may be used if additional calories are needed, as MCT absorption depends on minimal amounts of pancreatic enzymes. If steatorrhoea is controlled, fat-soluble vitamins do not need to be prescribed.

Pancreatic enzyme supplements should be taken with meals. As up to 10 tablets a day may be needed to control symptoms, compliance is often poor. Because some preparations are inactivated at a low pH, acid-suppression therapy is also usually given. Creon is an enteric-coated preparation which is released in the distal duodenum and thus does not require concomitant acid-suppression therapy.

The response to treatment can be assessed by an improvement in steatorrhoea, weight gain and a reduction in the 24-hour faecal fat excretion. For those patients who are chronically debilitated, or at times of severe complications, total parenteral feeding should be considered.

3. *Diabetes.* Insulin is usually needed, but the insulin requirements are usually low due to a concomitant lack of glucagon. Diabetic control is frequently difficult, and hypoglycaemia is a common problem and is often unpredictable.

Complications

1. Pseudocysts. These are collections of pancreatic secretions surrounded by fibrous walls of granulation tissue. They develop in approximately 10% of those with chronic pancreatitis and in most cases are in the body or tail of the gland. Most are asymptomatic and resolve spontaneously. Complications include rupture, haemorrhage into a cyst (which may be fatal) and infection. Distal pancreatectomy is indicated for large symptomatic cysts in the tail of the pancreas. External drainage may be achieved surgically, or percutaneously under radiological guidance. Internal drainage is either performed surgically or endoscopically. The surgical procedure depends on the site of the cyst and involves establishing a communication between the cyst and stomach, duodenum or small bowel. Endoscopic techniques are available to place a cystoenteric stent, to drain the cyst directly into the stomach.

2. Pancreatic duct strictures and stones. These cause stasis resulting in repeated acute attacks. Endoscopic balloon dilatation of strictures and extracorporeal shock-wave lithotripsy of calculi are possible therapeutic measures in referral centres.

3. Pancreatic ascites. Pancreatic fluid may leak into the peritoneal cavity from a ruptured duct or pseudocyst. The diagnosis is made with the finding of a high ascitic amylase and protein content. Treatment involves the use of diuretics and possibly octreotide. Therapeutic paracentesis is an option. ERCP-placed transpapillary stents to bridge ductal leaks is an option, although experience is limited. Surgical procedures involve the anastomosis of a defunctionalized Roux-en-Y loop of jejunum to the site of the ductal rupture, or distal pancreatectomy if the ductal leak is in the tail of the pancreas.

4. Fistulation. A pleural effusion may form when pancreatic fluid tracks into the pleural space via a pancreatico–pleural fistula. The treatment is pleural aspiration. Fistulae to other adjacent sites are less common.

5. Common bile-duct obstruction. This is a relatively common problem in those with long-standing chronic pancreatitis. The cause is either chronic inflammation and fibrosis in the head of the gland or a pseudocyst. The obstruction may be relieved with an endoscopically placed stent at ERCP or with a surgical bypass procedure.

6. Portal hypertension. This is a rare complication and is due to splenic or portal vein thrombosis or compression from a fibrotic pancreas or pseudocyst. Venography or Doppler studies will help to distinguish it from cirrhotic portal hypertension. Surgical portal decompression is occasionally successful.

7. *Pancreatic cancer.* The risk of pancreatic cancer is slightly increased in those with chronic pancreatitis. An estimated 4% of such patients develop pancreatic cancer within 20 years of diagnosis.

Prognosis

The mortality rate approaches 50% within 20–25 years. Up to 20% of patients die from complications related to acute exacerbations, with the remaining deaths caused by trauma (including suicide), cirrhosis, malnutrition, drug dependence, infection or complications related to smoking.

Further reading

Mergener K, Baillie J. Chronic pancreatitis. *Lancet*, 1997; **350:** 1379–85.
Steer ML, Waxman I, Freedman S. Chronic pancreatitis. *New England Journal of Medicine*, 1995; **332(22):** 1482–90.

Related topic of interest

Carcinoma of the pancreas (p. 27)

CIRRHOSIS

Cirrhosis is a histological diagnosis implying irreversible liver damage: a diffuse process of fibrosis with intervening nodular regeneration, resulting from previous hepatocellular necrosis.

Classification

Three types are recognized:

- Macronodular cirrhosis: characterized by fibrous septa and nodules of varying size, with islands of normal, regenerating tissue within the larger nodules.
- Micronodular cirrhosis: characterized by thick regular septa separating small, uniform nodules, often with marked fatty change. This type is seen in cases with an impaired capacity for regrowth (e.g. alcoholism, malnutrition, old age).
- Mixed micro- and macronodular cirrhosis: regeneration in micronodular cirrhosis results in macronodular change, and a mixed picture.

Causes

- Chronic hepatitis B (with or without delta), chronic hepatitis C infection and alcohol account for 70% of cases.
- Other causes are numerous and include autoimmune diseases (e.g. primary biliary cirrhosis, chronic autoimmune hepatitis), metabolic diseases (e.g. haemochromatosis, Wilson's disease, α_1-antitrypsin deficiency, galactosaemia), hepatic venous outflow obstruction (e.g. Budd–Chiari syndrome, right heart failure, veno-occlusive disease), drugs (e.g. methotrexate, amiodarone), cholestasis (e.g. sclerosing cholangitis, cystic fibrosis, prolonged parenteral nutrition).
- In the UK, 10% of cases have no obvious cause ('cryptogenic cirrhosis'). With more accurate diagnostic tests, this proportion seems to be falling.

Clinical features

Patients with *compensated cirrhosis* have deranged liver enzymes and may be asymptomatic or present with vague symptoms of fatigue or anorexia. Examination may reveal muscle wasting, palmar erythema, finger clubbing, spider naevi, purpura, pedal oedema, leuconychia, gynaecomastia, testicular atrophy, parotid enlargement, Dupuytren's contracture, hepatosplenomegaly and ascites. Such patients may die of other unrelated causes, or progress to hepatocellular failure. The rate of progression depends upon the cause of cirrhosis and is often difficult to predict.

Decompensated cirrhosis manifests with features of hepatocellular failure and/or portal hypertension. Apart from the clinical findings in those with compensated cirrhosis, patients may also have jaundice, foetor hepaticus, asterixis, hepatic encephalopathy, ascites, coagulopathy or variceal bleeding.

1. Laboratory investigations. Biochemical tests may be normal, or show variable elevations in liver enzymes, raised bilirubin and gamma globulins. The synthetic ability of the liver is assessed by the serum albumin and PT. A mild, normochromic, normocytic anaemia and reduced leucocyte and platelet counts ('hypersplenism') are also commonly found. The alpha-fetoprotein level may be mildly elevated in the absence of a hepatocellular carcinoma.

Initial laboratory investigations to detect the underlying cause include viral hepatitis serology, an autoantibody screen, serum ferritin, transferrin and iron binding capacity, serum caeruloplasmin, serum and urine copper measurements and α_1-antitrypsin level.

2. Liver biopsy. Cirrhosis can only accurately be diagnosed with a liver biopsy. The percutaneous approach is acceptable for those with no ascites, a platelet count of $>100 \times 10^9/l$, no focal lesion requiring targetting, no evidence of biliary obstruction on ultrasound scan and a normal PT. Those with a mildly prolonged PT should be treated with 2–4 units of fresh frozen plasma immediately prior to the procedure. A 'plugged' biopsy under radiological control is advisable in such circumstances. Ultrasound-guided biopsies should also be used if a focal lesion is present and if the procedure does not appear to be straightforward (e.g. an obese patient, or a patient with a poor respiratory function). Those with a significant coagulopathy or ascites should have a transjugular biopsy.

3. Imaging studies. An ultrasound scan may show ascites and changes suggestive of cirrhosis – irregular hyperechoic areas and nodules. Doppler studies should be performed to assess the patency of the portal and hepatic veins.

A CT scan provides an objective record of the appearance and size of the liver. The newer techniques of spiral CT and MRI provide more accurate images, and are especially useful if a hepatoma is suspected within a diffusely cirrhotic liver.

Assessment of hepatocellular function – other associations

- Malnutrition. This is multifactorial, and is greatest in those with alcoholic cirrhosis and those with Child's grade C (see below). Contributing factors include: reduced fat stores and total body protein turnover; increased basal metabolic rate; reduced hepatic bile salt secretion resulting in steatorrhoea; small bowel bacterial overgrowth and chronic relapsing pancreatitis (common in alcoholics).
- Peptic ulceration. This is usually duodenal ulceration and is often asymptomatic.

- Infections. Septicaemia is a frequent cause of deterioration and death in end-stage disease. Increased susceptibility is partly due to reduced leucocyte phagocytic activity, increased intestinal permeability to microorganisms, porto-systemic shunts and the risks of spontaneous bacterial peritonitis.
- Renal effects. Cortical blood flow is reduced in cirrhosis, and is further reduced in times of hypovolaemia (e.g. due to shock, over-vigorous diuresis, large volume ascitic drainage with inadequate i.v. colloid cover). These changes may predispose to the hepato-renal syndrome.

Classification

The Pugh–Child's classification is used to grade hepatocellular function in cirrhosis. It is most useful in predicting the likelihood of bleeding from oesophageal varices, and in comparing outcomes from transplant surgery in groups of patients. It is relatively insensitive in predicting the prognosis in an individual patient. Three groups are described, A–C, in increasing order of severity. The measurements used to score these groups are shown in *Table 1*.

Table 1. Measurements used to score Pugh–Child's classification

Measurement	Points scored		
	1	2	3
Bilirubin (μmol)[a]	<35	35–50	>50
Albumin (g/l)	>35	28–35	<28
Ascites	None	Slight	Moderate
Encephalopathy	Absent	Grade I–II	Grade III–IV
Prothrombin time (secs prolonged)	1–4	4–6	>6

[a] Note: in primary biliary cirrhosis, bilirubin is scored at <70 = 1; 70–170 = 2; >170 = 3.

The scores for the five variables are added together, and three overall classes derived: a score of 5–6 = 'A'; score 7–9 = 'B'; score >10 = 'C'.

Treatment

Although cirrhosis is irreversible, it is not necessarily progressive. In alcoholic cirrhosis, if the patient becomes totally abstinent, a Child's A classification carries an excellent prognosis. Abstinence from alcohol should also be aimed for in those with cirrhosis from other causes.

Those with malnutrition will require enteral supplements, and sometimes parenteral nutrition (e.g. prior to liver transplantation). A diet containing 1 g of protein/kg bodyweight/day is usually adequate. This may need to be increased in those with malnutrition and reduced in those at risk of hepatic encephalopathy. Those with ascites and oedema should be recommended a salt-restricted diet.

Potentially hepatotoxic drugs should be avoided, as well as those which may precipitate hepatic encephalopathy.

Antifibrotic drugs aimed at switching off collagen synthesis (e.g. colchicine, corticosteroids, γ-interferon) are promising, but have not yet become standard treatment.

All operations in cirrhotic patients carry a high risk and should be avoided if possible. The operative mortality depends on the Child's grade: grade A has 10% mortality; grade B, 30% mortality; and grade C, 75% mortality.

Further specific treatment depends upon the underlying cause and the specific complications.

Prognosis

This depends on the aetiology, clinical severity (e.g. Child's classification), histological severity and options for treatment (e.g. antiviral agents). Jaundice, coagulopathy, refractory ascites and bacterial peritonitis are ominous clinical signs. Decompensation in the absence of a treatable cause, hyponatraemia (in the absence of diuretic therapy) and hypoalbuminaemia are also all poor prognostic features. Serum transaminase levels have no bearing on prognosis. Patients with alcoholic cirrhosis and Child's A grade have a 5-year survival of 80–90% if abstinent, and 30% if they continue drinking.

Further reading

Friedman SL. The cellular basis of hepatic fibrosis: mechanisms and treatment strategies. *New England Journal of Medicine*, 1993; **328:** 1828.

Related topics of interest

Ascites (p. 14)
Hepatic tumours (p. 150)
Portal hypertension (p. 223)
Transplantation – liver (p. 254)

COELIAC DISEASE

Coeliac disease (CD) is a chronic inflammatory condition of the small intestinal mucosa (predominantly the proximal small intestine) that impairs nutrient absorption, and improves after gluten is withdrawn from the diet. Synonyms include 'coeliac sprue', 'non-tropical sprue' and 'gluten sensitive enteropathy'. Gluten is a group of proteins found in wheat; α-gliadin is one of the toxic subfractions. Similar proteins in barley and rye cause intestinal damage, while oat grains *may* be tolerated, in patients with coeliac disease. The mechanism by which the host's immune response to gluten damages the mucosa is unknown.

Incidence and epidemiology

The prevalence in the UK is 1 in 1000 to 1 in 1500 (the highest rate is 1 in 300, found in western Ireland). High rates of CD have also been found in Scandinavia (particularly Norway) and in northern Italy. There is a familial inheritance in first-degree relatives of about 10%.

Clinical features

The disease may present at any age with a multitude of manifestations. The severity of the disease seems to depend on the length of small intestine that is damaged. The symptoms may be very subtle and extra-intestinal symptoms often predominate. The commonest mode of presentation in the adult is iron-deficiency anaemia. Gross malabsorption and weight loss is now rare.

The age at diagnosis in adults follows two peaks – one in the third decade and one in the fifth and sixth decades. Symptoms may be provoked by infection, pregnancy or surgery. Specific features at diagnosis include:

- General lassitude (in 80–90%).
- Diarrhoea (75–80%). This may be infrequent or absent. Flatulence and bloating are often associated. Constipation may coexist with CD. Steatorrhoea, although not uncommon in the past, is nowadays rare.
- Weight loss.
- Nutritional deficiencies. 85% have asymptomatic iron or folate deficiency. Anaemia (particularily iron-deficiency) may be the only indication of CD. Other nutritional deficiencies include vitamin D deficiency (producing bone pain, osteoporosis, tetany, myopathy). Vitamin K deficiency occurs in up to 10%.
- Hyposplenism (Howell–Jolly bodies and target cells) is found in half of adult patients at diagnosis.
- Dermatitis herpetiformis (see below).
- Other features include menstrual irregularities, psychological disturbances, oral aphthous ulceration and (rarely) finger clubbing.

| Investigations | *Diagnostic tests.* An endoscopic biopsy from the distal duodenum (or ideally, the proximal jejunum with the use of a push-enteroscope) is mandatory to establish the diagnosis. Subsequent gluten challenge is not necessary for adult patients. Characteristic histological findings include villous atrophy, crypt hyperplasia, chronic inflammatory cell infiltration of the lamina propria and intra-epithelial lymphocyte infiltration. Confusion may occur if the changes are mild, and in the occasional case when villous atrophy is patchy. Villi are normally relatively flattened in the duodenal bulb (and especially so in duodenal ulcer disease), and an inadvertent biopsy may produce a false positive result. Biopsies should be repeated after 6 months on a gluten-free diet (GFD) to confirm the histological response.

Serological studies for antibodies to gliadin and endomysium are used to support the diagnosis, for screening purposes, and to monitor progress (levels fall with treatment). IgG and IgA anti-gliadin antibodies are easily measured and are sensitive (present in 90% of those with untreated disease) but not specific. IgA anti-endomysial antibody has a greater specificity (approaching 100%) and a sensitivity of 90–95%. Anti-endomysial antibody may be falsely negative in those with an IgA deficiency, which occasionally coexists with CD. |
| Other investigations | The following tests should be carried out in all cases: full blood count, vitamin B_{12}, red blood cell folate, iron, serum albumin, calcium and alkaline phosphatase. These should be repeated at annual follow-up and during pregnancy. Bone densitometry testing should be performed periodically.

The following are indicative of generalized intestinal malabsorption and may be found in CD: reduced fat-soluble vitamin levels (i.e. A, D and E as measured directly, and K as measured by a prolonged PT); low serum cholesterol, magnesium, potassium and phosphate; increased faecal fat excretion.

Small bowel barium studies may sometimes be required to exclude other causes of malabsorption (e.g. ileal Crohn's disease or jejunal diverticulosis) and to detect complications of CD (e.g. strictures and small-bowel lymphoma). |
| Differential diagnosis | Other causes of villous atrophy in adults are: |

- *Giardia lamblia* infection.
- Bacterial overgrowth.
- Acute viral enteritis.
- Tropical sprue.
- Human immunodeficiency virus (HIV) enteropathy.
- Small-bowel vasculitis.
- Primary lymphoma of the small intestine.

- Whipple's disease.
- NSAIDs.
- Radiation.
- Hypogammaglobulinaemia.
- Starvation.
- Gastrinoma.

Treatment

1. Gluten-free diet. An absolute GFD is the cornerstone of treatment. This involves the dietary exclusion of wheat, rye and barley (small amounts of oats are probably not toxic in the adult form of the disease). Strict adherence to the diet reduces the risk of complications (see below), and therefore must be continued for life.

Seventy percent of patients respond promptly to a GFD (usually within days to weeks), while histological improvement takes 3–12 months or more. Follow-up should be life long, with particular attention being made in times of increased nutritional demand (e.g. during emotional and physical stress and pregnancy).

2. Nutritional supplementation. Calcium and vitamin D should be given to those with osteopaenia. Iron, folic acid and magnesium should be replaced if any signs of deficiency are evident. Pregnancy is a particularly vulnerable time for nutritional deficiencies to occur, and folic acid levels in particular should be closely monitored. Vitamin B_{12} deficiency is uncommon in CD, as the disease predominantly affects the proximal small intestine.

A GFD is poor in fibre and may exacerbate constipation and symptoms of the irritable bowel syndrome. Fybogel is a suitable gluten-free fibre supplement.

Poor responders

If there is no clinical or histological improvement after 6 months:

- Assess compliance with a careful dietary history. Poor compliance is by far the commonest cause of persistent symptoms, and some people are exquisitely sensitive to the smallest amount of gluten.
- Confirm the diagnosis by reviewing the original histology and serology and by repeating the biopsies.
- Coincident or associated diseases must be excluded:
  Undiagnosed nutritional deficiencies should be sought and treated.
  Hypolactasia (due to mucosal atrophy) may be a cause, thus dairy products should be excluded from the diet for a trial period of 4 weeks.
  Giardiasis should be excluded by examination of a jejunal aspiration – and even if *Giardia lamblia* are not

found, a therapeutic trial of a single dose of tinidazole (2 g) could be given.

Hypogammaglobulinaemia and Addison's disease should be excluded.

Small-bowel lymphoma, Crohn's disease and jejunal diverticulosis should be excluded with a barium meal and follow-through.

Pancreatic exocrine deficiency is occasionally associated – usually only in those with longstanding malabsorption – and can be detected with a PABA test or pancrelauryl breath test.

Refractory disease

Some patients do not respond to a strict GFD ('refractory sprue'). Some respond to corticosteroids (prednisolone up to 60 mg/day may be needed) and immunosuppressants (usually azathioprine). A jejunal biopsy should be repeated after 3 months, and if no improvement has occurred, a referral to a specialist centre is advised.

Associated disorders and complications

1. Dermatitis herpetiformis. This intensely pruritic papulovesicular rash is mainly found on the elbows and buttocks. Immunofluorescent staining of a biopsy from uninvolved skin reveals IgA deposits in the upper dermis. Mucosal lesions in the small intestine, indistinguishable from coeliac disease, are almost invariably found. Both the intestinal lesions and the rash respond to a GFD. Dapsone may be used to treat the skin lesions but it does not heal the bowel pathology. Side-effects include a dose-dependent haemolytic anaemia, methaemoglobinaemia and headache.

2. Malignant lymphoma of the small intestine. Small-intestinal T-cell lymphoma is reported in 5–10% of known (mostly older) cases (the true incidence is probably lower as many cases of CD remain undiagnosed in the general population). The risk is reduced by the adherence to a strict GFD.

The commonest presentation is the return of diarrhoea, weight loss and lassitude in a patient with treated CD. It should also be rigorously excluded in those who fail to respond to a GFD. Abdominal pain, intestinal bleeding and fever are other suggestive symptoms.

The standard investigations of small-bowel barium studies and standard jejunal biopsy often have a low yield. A CT or MRI scan of the abdomen may reveal a thickened small-bowel wall and intra-abdominal lymphadenopathy. Biopsy of a peripheral lymph node or bone marrow, or radiologically guided liver or abdominal lymph node biopsy will confirm the diagnosis. Small-bowel push-enteroscopy, if available, will allow direct visualization and serial biopsies of the small intestine.

Laparotomy (or laparoscopy) and biopsies of lymph nodes, liver and full-thickness samples of the small intestine are often needed to obtain a definitive diagnosis.

Treatment is difficult and involves local resection, radiotherapy and chemotherapy.

3. Other malignancies. There is a twofold increased risk overall for neoplasia at all sites, but the relative risk is greatest by far for gastrointestinal malignancies. Adenocarcinoma is more common anywhere in the gastrointestinal tract, and in the small bowel usually produces non-specific symptoms, thus the disease has usually metastasized by the time of diagnosis. Treatment is surgical with adjuvant chemotherapy, but the prognosis is poor. Extra-intestinal lymphoma and carcinomas of the oropharynx and breast occur with increased incidence.

4. Chronic ulcerative enteritis (ulcerative jejunoileitis). This is a rare complication of CD in which small intestinal ulceration and stricturing presents as a protein-losing enteropathy, or with symptoms of severe refractory CD. Medical treatment is often unrewarding and early surgical resection is indicated if symptoms do not settle on a GFD.

5. Other diseases. Numerous other diseases have been associated with CD, some of which are listed below.

- Neurological disorders (spinocerebellar degeneration, peripheral neuropathy, epilepsy with cerebral calcification).
- Autoimmune diseases (insulin-dependent diabetes, thyrotoxicosis, Addison's disease).
- Gastrointestinal diseases (ulcerative colitis, primary biliary cirrhosis, primary sclerosing cholangitis).
- Miscellaneous (selective IgA deficiency, IgA mesangial nephropathy, rheumatoid arthritis).

Screening

The prevalence of asymptomatic CD is high in the general population, and since it is known that the strict adherence to a GFD reduces the incidence of complications, it is recommended that those at risk of CD should be screened with anti-gliandin and anti-endomysial antibody titres. These include first-degree relatives of those with CD (who have an inheritance of CD of around 10%), and those with type I diabetes, iron-deficiency anaemia, unexplained neurological disease and recurrent aphthous stomatitis.

Prognosis

Most patients who adhere to a GFD remain well and ultimately die of unrelated causes. The overall mortality rate is, however, increased owing to the number of associated disorders outlined above. The exact magnitude is controversial.

Useful address	The Coeliac Society of the UK
	PO Box 220
	High Wycombe
	Bucks HP11 2HY
	Tel: 01494 437278

Further reading

British Society of Gastroenterology. Guidelines for the management of patients with coeliac disease. September 1996.
Howdle PD (ed). Coeliac disease. *Bailliere's Clinical Gastroenterology*, 1995; **9(2):** 191–370.
Trier JS. Celiac sprue. *New England Journal of Medicine*, 1991; **325(24):** 1709–19.

Related topics of interest

Malabsorption (p. 189)
Tumours of the small intestine (p. 261)

COLITIS – NON-SPECIFIC

Lymphocytic colitis

This is a rare disease predominantly affecting women over the age of 60. Patients present with chronic watery diarrhoea and cramping abdominal discomfort. Weight loss is usually mild and other symptoms of inflammatory bowel disease, including bloody diarrhoea, fever and acute exacerbations, are typically absent. The disease usually runs a benign course and spontaneous remissions may occur.

An immune aetiology is likely as the disease is associated with an increased frequency of the human leucocyte antigen (HLA) A1 genotype, and an association with coeliac disease, seronegative arthritis and Raynaud's disease is described.

Routine blood tests, including inflammatory markers, are normal. Stool microscopy for blood, leucocytes and pathogens are negative. Colonoscopy appears macroscopically normal. The diagnosis is made on serial biopsies of the colon, which emphasizes the need to take biopsies on colonoscopy even if the mucosa appears normal. Characteristically, a prominent epithelial lymphocytic infiltration is seen, with otherwise normal mucosal architecture (hence the old term 'microscopic colitis'). Other causes of chronic diarrhoea (see p. 81), including coeliac disease and high sorbitol intake, should always be excluded. It is possible that many cases are being missed at present and are possibly being incorrectly labelled as irritable bowel syndrome.

No specific treatment has been agreed upon, although up to 50% of patients respond to sulphasalazine, at a starting dose of 1 g twice daily. Prednisolone is useful to control exacerbations, and should be used in the same regimen as for Crohn's disease. Cholestyramine (1–2 g twice daily before meals) or metronidazole have been used empirically with variable success, and are acceptable add-in therapies if needed.

Collagenous colitis

This condition also occurs mainly in middle-aged women and runs a similar clinical course to lymphocytic colitis. An immune aetiology is also implicated, and reports have described histological progression from lymphocytic colitis to collagenous colitis, suggesting that they may be different manifestations of the same disease process. Collagenous colitis, unlike lymphocytic colitis, may be associated with long-term use of NSAIDs. A peripheral arthritis is associated in 7% cases. No HLA association is described.

Like lymphocytic colitis, routine blood tests are normal and, although the colonic mucosa appears normal on colonoscopy, the diagnosis is made histologically. The finding of a patchy collagen layer in the subepithelial region, greater than 10 μm wide (normally about 3 μm), is characteristic. An intra-epithelial lymphocytic infiltration (as with lymphocytic colitis) is also commonly seen.

Management involves stopping any NSAIDs and excluding CD and other causes of chronic watery diarrhoea. Treatment and response to treatment is the same as for lymphocytic colitis.

Diversion colitis

This occurs in the defunctioned loop of colon after the formation of a more proximal colostomy. The condition is relatively common and presents as a mucus discharge. Sigmoidoscopy may reveal generalized mucosal hyperaemia with mucosal lymphoid follicles. Biopsies reveal a lymphocytic infiltrate in the lamina propria with prominent lymphoid follicular hyperplasia. Minimal crypt distortion and goblet cell depletion are also seen. The features are similar to mild ulcerative colitis.

Treatment with short-chain fatty acid enemas (e.g. sodium butyrate) is usually effective. The rationale for this is that normal colonic epithelium utilizes butyrate, a short-chain fatty acid produced by bacterial digestion of dietary fibre, as its principal energy source. Replacement of this, which is deficient in a defunctioned colon, restores this energy source. As with ulcerative colitis, 5-aminosalicylic acid (5-ASA) enemas are also effective. The condition resolves when the colon is re-joined.

Pouchitis

Up to 40% of patients with ulcerative colitis treated with a colectomy and ileo–anal pouch anastamosis experience inflammation of the pouch reservoir ('pouchitis'), with symptoms similar to an exacerbation of proctitis. This is more common in patients who have experienced extracolonic manifestations, and possibly represents a form of recurrent ulcerative colitis of the pouch ileal cells transformed by colonic metaplasia. Other causes which should be sought and treated include a local gastroenteric infection, postoperative sepsis and mechanical outlet obstruction of the pouch.

Treatment is initially with metronidazole (400 mg three times daily), which usually leads to a reduction in the frequency of evacuation. Topical and systemic steroids and 5-ASA preparations are also often effective. Most patients experience infrequent relapses; however, about 5% have chronic symptoms necessitating maintenance therapy.

Further reading

Stampfl DA, Friedman LS. Collagenous colitis. Pathophysiological considerations. *Digestive Disease and Science*, 1991; **36(6):** 705–11.

Mills LR, Schuman BM, Thompson WO. Lymphocytic colitis. A definable clinical and histological diagnosis. *Digestive Disease and Science*, 1993; **38(6):** 1147–51.

Related topic of interest

Ulcerative colitis – background and clinical features (p. 265)
Ulcerative colitis – medical and surgical management (p. 269)

COLONIC POLYPS

The term 'polyp' describes any elevation above the mucosal surface. They can be either sessile or pedunculated and may be single or multiple. They are broadly categorized, histologically, as either neoplastic (benign or malignant) or non-neoplastic. Neoplastic polyps are usually larger with a more erythematous surface than non-neoplastic polyps; however, these macroscopic features are unreliable and all polyps should be biopsied.

Non-neoplastic polyps

These can be divided into four groups.

Metaplastic (hyperplastic) polyps
These are mainly found in the rectum, and are the commonest type of rectal polyp overall. The incidence increases with age. They are usually small (<5 mm), sessile and are often multiple in the elderly. Characteristic histological features distinguish them from neoplastic polyps, and they have no malignant potential.

Inflammatory polyps
These are tags of normal mucosa (occasionally containing granulation tissue) that arise in the setting of colitis. They are either active (as islands of mucosa between areas of ulceration) or quiescent. Although they may appear sinister, they are benign and have no malignant potential.

Lymphoid polyps are another form of inflammatory polyp. They may be single (usually in the rectum of young adults) or multiple (diffuse lymphoid hyperplasia, which is a normal finding in children), and may be seen in adults following an episode of infective colitis.

Hamartomatous polyps
These are focal, disorganized proliferations of normal tissue. These polyps are those found in the Peutz–Jeghers syndrome and juvenile polyposis (see 'Hereditary neoplastic syndromes of the intestine' (p. 166)). Juvenile polyps are pedunculated, and present in childhood (occasionally in adults) with rectal bleeding, intussusception or prolapse through the anus. They may be multiple and the whole colon should be examined if one is found distally. They characteristically contain cystic inclusions of mucus, and are sometimes called mucus retention polyps. Hamartomatous polyps very occasionally develop areas of dysplasia within a single polyp, which can lead to sporadic small or large bowel cancer.

Miscellaneous polyps
Lipomas are usually seen in the right colon as submucosal rounded elevations with a regular, shiny surface. The appearance is characteristic and biopsy confirms the diagnosis. They have no malignant potential.

Endometriosis and leiomyomas occasionally present as polypoid lesions.

Neoplastic polyps (adenomas)

These are the commonest colonic polyps in patients of >55 years of age. They are classified as either tubular, villous or tubulo-villous. Tubular adenomas are the commonest, and usually have a stalk with a head containing branching glands lined by dysplastic epithelium. Villous adenomas are usually sessile and larger, with enlarged, elongated surface crypts covered by dysplastic epithelium. Tubulo-villous adenomas have features of both and account for about one-quarter of adenomas.

Overall, about 10% of colonic adenomas progress to carcinomas. The propensity to develop malignant change is related to the degree of dysplasia (graded as mild, moderate or severe), the type of adenoma (villous adenomas being the most likely and tubular adenomas the least) and size (increasing size over 1 cm raises the risk of malignant change). Carcinoma is diagnosed when the dysplastic epithelial cells invade across the muscularis mucosa.

Clinical features Most polyps are detected incidentally during investigations for other symptoms, and are asymptomatic. Larger polyps may cause overt rectal bleeding or iron-deficiency anaemia. Large villous adenomas of the rectum may occasionally cause mucoid diarrhoea and hypokalaemia.

Management Most patients with no family history of colorectal polyps or cancer, who are found to have polyps on barium enema or sigmoidoscopy, should be offered a total colonoscopy. Pedunculated polyps are snared and removed, and sessile polyps can be biopsied and destroyed by electrocoagulation (this may require several sessions for larger polyps). Histological assessment can then be made of the type of polyp, degree of dysplasia and whether the resection was complete or incomplete (i.e. whether the stalk was clear of dysplastic cells or not).

Those with adenomas >2 cm in size should undergo follow-up colonoscopy in 3–6 months to assess the completeness of the resection. Residual polyps should be removed and if, after two to three examinations, resection is incomplete, surgical removal should be considered.

Malignant polyps which are completely excised and not poorly differentiated should be reassessed 3 months later to exclude residual abnormal tissue. Malignant polyps other than these should be considered for surgical resection. Patients who are a poor operative risk should be offered a local excision.

Surveillance Follow-up surveillance after colonoscopic removal of polyps should be individualized according to the type and number of polyps. After one normal colonoscopy at 3 years, the interval may be increased to 5 years. There is, however, no universal agreement as to the optimum frequency and timing of colono-scopic follow-up.

Further reading

Bond JH. Polyp guideline: diagnosis, treatment, and surveillance for patients with non-familial colorectal polyps. *Annals of Internal Medicine*, 1993; **119:** 836–43.

Related topic of interest

Colorectal cancer and screening (p. 55)

COLORECTAL CANCER AND SCREENING

Colorectal cancer

Background

Colorectal cancer is the second most common cause of death from malignant disease in the Western world. In the UK, 20 000 people die from this disease each year. The vast majority of colonic cancer originates from adenomatous polyps, and the progression from polyp to cancer probably takes 10–15 years. The major exception to this are patients who develop cancer associated with long-standing inflammatory bowel disease, where the cancer develops from an area of dysplastic epithelium.

Risk factors and pathogenesis

Patients with familial adenomatous polyposis (FAP) carry a 100% lifetime risk of colorectal cancer (see p. 166). Most patients with FAP if untreated would be dead from colonic cancer by their late thirties. Hereditary non-polyposis colorectal cancer (HNPCC) is a dominantly inherited condition which results in predominantly right-sided cancers, which often become manifest at a relatively young age (thirties to forties). Most patients with colorectal cancer, however, have 'sporadic' disease. Sporadic colorectal cancer also has a genetic element to it. Approximately 25% of patients with colorectal cancer have a positive family history.

The relative risk of developing colorectal cancer is greater the larger the number of relatives affected. In addition, the closer the relationship and the younger the age at diagnosis, the greater is the risk. *Table 1* gives a rough guide to the lifetime risk of colorectal cancer.

Table 1. Lifetime risks for colorectal cancer

Family history	Lifetime risk
None	1:50
One first-degree relative >45 years	1:18
One first-degree relative <45 years	1:10
Two first-degree relatives	1:6

Patients with inflammatory bowel disease are also at increased risk of developing colorectal cancer. This was originally described in patients with ulcerative colitis. In patients with ulcerative colitis, which affects the whole colon, the risk of developing colorectal cancer is 5–10% at 20 years. Recent data suggest the same may be true for patients with colonic Crohn's disease.

The molecular mechanisms involved in the pathogenesis of colorectal cancer are slowly emerging. Current work has focused on the role of tumour suppresser genes such as *p53*, which appear to be inactive in patients with colorectal cancer. Furthermore, the oncogenes K-*ras* and c-*myc* are activated. These disturbances at the molecular level impair control of epithelial growth and repair, ultimately leading to carcinogenesis.

Clinical features

Colorectal carcinoma presents in several different ways:

- Iron deficiency anaemia.
- Change in bowel habit.
- Abdominal pain.
- Rectal bleeding.
- As a surgical emergency:
    Obstruction.
    Lower gastrointestinal haemorrhage.
    Perforation (rare).

Rectal cancers tend to present relatively early with rectal bleeding, mucus discharge, frequency and urgency. Cancers further round the colon, and particularly in the right side of the colon, tend to present later with abdominal pain and anaemia.

Clinical examination should always include a rectal examination, as a significant proportion of rectal cancers may be detected with the finger. Other features to look for include:

- Palpable mass.
- Signs of iron deficiency anaemia.
- Hepatomegaly (disseminated disease).
- Local lymph node involvement.

Colonic cancer is a slowly growing cancer and in the early stages of the disease the symptoms are non-specific and clinical examination is normal. All too often this leads to a delay in diagnosis which could adversely affect the prognosis. It is important to keep a high index of suspicion for this cancer and in particular:

- Never assume rectal bleeding is due to piles until proven otherwise.
- Always do a PR examination.
- A significant change in bowel habit in a patient over the age of 40 always requires investigation.
- Always investigate the colon in a patient with iron deficiency anaemia, unless there is a *very* good reason not to.

Investigations

The basic tools used to investigate patients for colorectal cancer are:

- The finger (PR examination).
- Rigid sigmoidoscopy.

- Flexible sigmoidoscopy.
- Barium enema.
- Colonoscopy.

It is important whichever combination of these techniques is used that the whole of the colon is adequately visualized. Different combinations of these investigations have differing sensitivities and specificities for the diagnosis of colorectal cancer, all of which are operator dependent. However, the best technique, particularly in the patient with overt rectal bleeding, is colonoscopy by an expert. The sensitivity and specificity of this test under these circumstances is >95%. Once the diagnosis is established, an ultrasound or CT will help to stage the disease. CT is the superior technique. The place of spiral CT, spiral CT with pneumocolon and virtual colonoscopy with spiral CT remains to be established.

Treatment

1. Surgery. The cornerstone of treatment is surgical excision. The basic principles of surgery in colorectal cancer include:

- Removal of the tumour with wide excision margins.
- Removal of related vascular and lymphatic fields.
- Preservation of anal sphincter where possible (use of staple guns).
- Avoidance of a stoma where possible.

Approximately 80% of patients have surgery in the hope of a cure.

2. Radiotherapy. Patients with rectal cancer should be given preoperative radiotherapy. There is evidence that this reduces the recurrence rate and improves survival from colorectal cancer. Postoperative radiotherapy in patients with rectal cancer reduces local recurrence but does not improve survival. Furthermore, postoperative radiotherapy causes more long-term morbidity than a brief 1-week course of preoperative radiotherapy.

In patients with locally advanced rectal cancer, radiotherapy is a highly effective palliative tool. Such patients often have very distressing symptoms. Good symptom control can also be achieved using laser ablation.

3. Chemotherapy. Adjuvant chemotherapy is only helpful in patients with Dukes' stage C disease. Treatment with 5-fluorouracil (5FU)/folinic acid for 6 months achieves about a 30% reduction in mortality in this group. The role of adjuvant chemotherapy in patients with Dukes' stage B disease remains under investigation.

In patients with advanced or recurrent disease, palliative treatment with 5FU and methotrexate or folinic acid has been shown to prolong survival by several months. This is most effective when given by continuous infusion rather than by bolus doses. Intra-arterial infusion into the hepatic artery in patients with liver metastases also prolongs survival.

Follow-up

Most patients who have had 'curative' surgery for colorectal cancer are offered follow-up. This includes a combination of the following:

- Colonoscopy.
- Serial CEA levels.
- Flexible sigmoidoscopy.
- Barium studies.
- CT scans.

There is no consensus as to the optimum nature, extent or frequency of follow-up and recent data suggest that intensive follow-up may have little discernible effect on survival. Most recurrences are discovered as a result of symptoms reported by patients. Most recurrences detected by follow-up surveillances are not amenable to curative treatment.

Prognosis

This has changed little in the past 30 years. For details, see *Table 2*.

Table 2. Prognosis for colorectal cancer

Disease	Prognosis	5-year survival (%)
Dukes' A	Tumour limited to bowel wall	95–100
Dukes' B	Penetration of bowel wall No nodes involved	65–75
Dukes' C	As B, with nodes involved	30–40
Dukes' D	Distant metastases	<1

When screening for colorectal cancer is introduced on a systematic basis, these figures should improve.

Screening for colorectal cancer

Population screening

The aim of population screening for colorectal cancer is to detect polyps before they become malignant and to detect cancers at an early stage when they are still curable (Dukes' A). For population screening to become a practicable proposition, any screening test will have to show a significant reduction in mortality from colorectal cancer, given the costs involved.

Two approaches to population screening for colorectal cancer have been the subject of considerable study over the last few years.

1. Faecal occult blood testing. Three large, long-term double-blind trials of population screening with faecal occult blood (FOB) tests for colorectal cancer have now been completed. All show a significant reduction in cancer mortality in the screened group, as shown in *Table 3* below.

Table 3. Population screening with FOB tests

Study	Compliance (%)	Reduction in mortality (%)
USA (Minnesota)	75	33
UK (Nottingham)	60	15
Denmark	67	18

Compliance was a problem in all three studies, and there were differences in the type of FOB test used and total colonoscopy rate. All showed a significant reduction in mortality; the highest figure of 33% was probably a result of the high colonoscopy rate in the study from the USA.

2. Flexible sigmoidoscopy. It has been suggested that a once-only flexible sigmoidoscopy at the age 55–60 may be an effective method of screening for colorectal cancer. The rationale is that most colorectal cancer occurs within reach of the flexible sigmoidoscope and patients who are identified as polyp formers can have more intensive surveillance. Non-controlled data suggest that this technique may reduce the death rate from colorectal cancer by as much as 60%. The problem with this technique, which is shared by FOB testing, is that a considerable number of cancers will still be missed.

Given the significant reduction in mortality in using either method for screening for colorectal cancer, it seems only a matter of time before screening becomes widespread. However, it is not yet clear which is the optimum approach. This is a complex issue and involves considerations such as:

- Cost.
- Compliance.
- Sensitivity.
- Specificity.

Screening high-risk groups

1. Hereditary non-polyposis cancer. Patients with a very strong family history, particularly in relatives at a young age or with right-sided colonic lesions, are often offered screening colonoscopy. The optimum timing and frequency of such examinations is unknown. A common practice is to offer colonoscopic screening every 5 years from the age of 25 years, when the risk is >1:10. There is no evidence that this reduces mortality.

2. Familial adenomatous polyposis. See p. 166.

3. Inflammatory bowel disease. There is no consensus about the optimum timing or frequency of colonoscopic screening in patients with inflammatory bowel disease. The data regarding its effectiveness in reducing cancer mortality is conflicting. A surveillance programme in common use for patients with long-standing pan-colitis is:

- Colonoscopy plus biopsy series at 10 years.
- Surveillance colonoscopy at 2–3-year intervals.
- Patients with severe dysplasia/frank carcinoma are offered colectomy.

Further reading

Anon. The management of colorectal cancer. *Effective Healthcare*, **3(6):** 1–12.

Hardcastle JD, Chamberlain JO, Robinson MHE *et al.* Randomized controlled trial of faecal-occult-blood screening for colorectal cancer. *Lancet*, 1996; **348:** 1472–7.

Kronborg O, Fenger C, Olsen J *et al.* Randomized study of screening for colorectal cancer with faecal-occult-blood test. *Lancet*, 1996; **348:** 1467–71.

Mandel JS, Bond JH, Church TR *et al.* Reducing mortality from colorectal cancer by screening for fecal occult blood. Minnesota Colon Cancer Control Study. *New England Journal of Medicine*, 1993; **328:** 1365–71.

Related topics of interest

CONSTIPATION

Constipation is a symptom, not a disease. The 'normal' frequency of bowel movements in western countries is very variable, ranging from about three a day to once every 3 days – some patients with even less frequent motions do not consider themselves to be constipated.

Definition

Constipation has no universal definition. One is: the presence of at least two of the following symptoms for at least 3 months:

- Stool frequency of less than two per week.
- Any of the following symptoms at least 25% of the time:
  Straining.
  Hard stools.
  Sensation of incomplete evacuation.

Prevalence

Constipation is the most common gastrointestinal complaint in the USA. In the UK, 2% of the population have fewer than two stools a week, and 12% experience straining at defecation. Constipation is commoner in women and in those over the age of 65.

Causes

1. Diet
- Insufficient fibre.
- Insufficient fluids.

2. Motility disorders
- Irritable bowel syndrome.
- Idiopathic slow transit.

3. Drugs
- Aluminium-containing antacids.
- Antidepressants.
- Anticholinergics.
- Iron.
- Barium.
- Opiates.
- Phenothiazines.
- Diuretics (causing dehydration and hypokalaemia).
- Calcium antagonists.

4. Metabolic diseases
- Diabetes (via an autonomic neuropathy).
- Hypercalcaemia.
- Hypothyroidism.
- Uraemia.
- Hypokalaemia.

5. Anorectal disease
- Anal fissure.
- Pelvic outlet obstruction – including the descending perineum syndrome (with or without mucosal prolapse and anismus).

6. *Intestinal obstruction*
- Colorectal carcinoma.
- Chronic intestinal pseudo-obstruction.
- Diverticular stricture.
- Aganglionosis – Hirschsprung's disease.

7. *Neurogenic conditions*
- Spinal cord injury.
- Amyotrophic lateral sclerosis.
- Cerebrovascular disease.
- Multiple sclerosis.
- Parkinson's disease.

Other predisposing factors are old age, poor mobility, inadequate toilet facilities, chronic stimulant laxative use (which produces damage to neural tissue in the bowel – the 'cathartic colon') and depression.

Approach to investigation

It is important to define what the patient means by constipation (i.e. infrequent stools, straining, or both). In all cases a thorough dietary and drug history is important. A positive family history may suggest a primary motility problem. A complicated obstetric history may suggest perineal pathology from neural damage.

Patients are evaluated according to their age, duration and severity of symptoms, and the presence or absence of 'warning' signs (e.g. weight loss, rectal bleeding, anaemia).

Examples are as follows:

- Middle-aged or elderly patients with a recent onset of constipation and no obvious cause should always be investigated for a possible colorectal carcinoma or diverticular stricture. Constipation with rectal bleeding should not automatically be assumed to be due to bleeding haemorrhoids or an anal fissure.
- Young patients with mild constipation and other symptoms consistent with the irritable bowel syndrome require reassurance and minimal investigations.
- Moderate to severe constipation since childhood suggests possible Hirschsprung's disease, megacolon or megarectum. Investigations include a barium enema, anorectal manometry and possibly a full-thickness rectal biopsy.
- Moderate to severe constipation in otherwise healthy young and middle-aged adults (usually in females) may indicate idiopathic slow-transit constipation or pelvic outlet obstruction.

Examination

A physical examination should be performed, including a rectal examination to determine the anal sphincter tone and to detect rectal masses, faecal loading, fissures, haemorrhoids or a rectal prolapse.

Investigations

1. Screening blood tests. These include a full blood count, electrolytes, glucose, calcium and thyroid function tests.

2. Sigmoidoscopy. A sigmoidoscopy is important to exclude a carcinoma of the rectum or distal sigmoid colon. Melanosis coli due to the chronic use of anthraquinone laxatives (e.g. senna, codanthrasate) may be evident.

3. Barium enema. This may show a colonic carcinoma, Hirschsprung's disease, megacolon/megarectum or redundant loops of large bowel. Megacolon and megarectum are defined as an ascending colon >8 cm in diameter, and a rectosigmoid colon >6.5 cm in diameter, respectively. Causes are chronic intestinal pseudo-obstruction, Hirschsprung's disease and idiopathic megacolon (which may be seen in any chronic constipation).

4. Colonic transit studies. These are useful for patients in whom no obvious cause can be found and who do not respond to simple therapies. Whilst on a high-fibre diet, the patient ingests 20 small radio-opaque markers, and a plain abdominal radiograph is performed 3 and 5 days later. Normal subjects pass their first marker within 3 days and 80% of the markers within 5 days. Patients are classified according to the following patterns:

- Normal transit time: the markers are expelled within the normal length of time. Constipation may have been due to a low-fibre diet, or psychological problems.
- Colonic inertia: markers are seen throughout the colon on day 5. This indicates a slow transit time which may be idiopathic, or secondary to a systemic disease or medication.
- Hindgut inertia: markers accumulate in the descending colon, indicating a segmental transit abnormality in the hindgut.
- Outlet obstruction: markers accumulate in the rectum and rectosigmoid. Causes include anismus (paradoxical contraction of the puborectalis muscle and external anal sphincter during defecation), descending perineum syndrome (± rectocoele) or internal anal sphincter dysfunction.
- Outlet obstruction may coexist with colonic or hindgut inertia.

The following tests used to assess anorectal function are usually only available in specialist centres.

5. Anorectal manometry. A balloon-tipped catheter is placed in the rectum, and rectal compliance and sensitivity is measured by inflating the balloon with increasing volumes of air. Pressure transducers simultaneously measure internal anal sphincter tone (which normally decreases with rectal distension and increases when the balloon is deflated). Anorectal manometry is usually used to assess anal sphincter tone in cases of faecal incontinence. Its main uses in constipation are:

- The diagnosis of adult Hirschsprung's disease and megarectum (secondary to aganglionosis), which are characterized by the absence of internal anal sphincter relaxation with rectal distension.
- Confirmation and treatment (by biofeedback conditioning) of anismus.

6. Electromyography. Needle electrodes are placed into the external sphincter and puborectalis muscle, and the myoelectric activity measured during attempted defecation. This test complements anorectal manometry, and is useful to assess pudendal nerve function in patients with faecal incontinence with or without constipation.

7. Barium defecography. This is usually used to assess women with suspected descending perineum syndrome. Such patients may have had a pudendal nerve injury during childbirth, and often complain of faecal incontinence with constipation. Tenesmus may be present, and the colonic transit study will show an outlet obstruction. During straining, the perineum is seen to descend, causing the rectal mucosa to prolapse (anterior or posterior rectocoele), which causes tenesmus and further straining. Such patients may benefit from a surgical repair.

Treatment

Treatment is initially aimed at the specific cause as outlined above. The majority of patients have a functional bowel disorder, and respond to simple dietary and lifestyle modification.

The patient's perceptions and expectations of normal bowel habit should be discussed. Patients should be counselled on the wide variability of normal frequency of bowel movements, and advised that a daily bowel movement is not necessary and often not a realistic goal. Patients should be encouraged to put a set time aside each day for defecation, and not to ignore a need to defecate. Physical activity should be increased, if appropriate. Those with proven slow-transit constipation may benefit from a prokinetic agent (e.g. cisapride, although this is an unlicensed indication). Cisapride may cause intestinal colic and can prolong the Q–T interval causing ventricular arrhythmias (particularly in combination with some antifungals – check the British National Formulary (BNF) for interactions if in doubt, as this could be fatal).

1. *Dietary advice.* Thirty grammes of dietary fibre and at least 1.5 l of fluid per day is recommended. Increased fibre intake should be introduced gradually, as those unaccustomed to such a diet may experience troublesome bloating and flatulence. A high-fibre diet may also increase abdominal symptoms in those with the irritable bowel syndrome. Patients should be advised that it may take several weeks for a high-fibre diet to work. Foods rich in fibre include wholemeal bread, cereals, fresh vegetables (beans, peas, green leafy vegetables) and fruit. Unprocessed coarse bran (1 tablespoon added to meals) can be added as a supplement, but many find it unpalatable. Ispaghula husk granules (e.g. Fybogel) are more convenient, but more expensive.

2. *Laxatives.* When needed, laxatives should be used as sparingly as possible, ideally on a temporary basis. Laxatives are contraindicated in bowel obstruction. Five groups are available:

- Bulk-forming laxatives – coarse bran, ispaghula husk (e.g. Fybogel), psillium (e.g. Metamucil) and sterculia (e.g. Normacol). All are useful first-line therapies, and should be used with an increased fluid intake.
- Osmotic laxatives, e.g. Lactulose. This is useful if a high-fibre diet and bulking agents have been ineffective. Although it is relatively expensive, it is useful in the elderly in whom it reduces the risk of urinary tract infections by altering the gut flora. Lactulose is also used to treat proximal constipation in distal ulcerative colitis. Lactulose produces an osmotic diarrhoea of low pH and discourages the proliferation of ammonia-producing organisms, and is thus used to prevent and treat hepatic encephalopathy.

  Macrogols (polyethylene glycols), e.g. Movicol, are a relatively new osmotic agent, useful for the short-term relief of chronic constipation.
- Saline agents – magnesium hydroxide (e.g. milk of magnesia), magnesium sulphate and sodium phosphate (e.g. Fleet phospho-soda, Fleet enema, phosphate enema). These are similar to osmotic agents, but also have some stimulant properties (see below). Magnesium sulphate (Epsom salts) is a useful first-line treatment in troublesome constipation. Enemas or suppositories act within an hour, and are useful for rapid relief. Sodium picosulphate with magnesium citrate (Picolax) is a more potent laxative and is used episodically in resistant constipation, and to prepare the bowel prior to an operation or procedure.

- Stimulant laxatives – senna (e.g. Senakot), bisacodyl (e.g. Dulcolax tablets or suppositories), castor oil, phenolphthalein (e.g. Ex-lax) and codanthrasate. These should be reserved for the temporary relief of severe constipation (e.g. those with neurological disorders), and as a bowel preparation prior to a procedure. Long-term use may damage the mucosal neural tissue, worsening the constipation ('cathartic megacolon').
- Emollients, lubricants and softeners, e.g. arachis oil enema, sodium docusate, glycerine suppository, mineral oil. These are used to soften and lubricate the stool to relieve rectal faecal impaction.

3. Treatment of descending perineum syndrome. Pelvic floor retraining, using exercises and biofeedback techniques to relax the puborectalis muscle and external sphincter (guided by anorectal manometry), is valuable in selected patients. Mucosal prolapse (e.g. rectocoele) can be treated with a submucosal injection of a sclerosant (e.g. phenol).

4. Surgery. In exceptional cases, intractable idiopathic slow-transit constipation may be treated by colectomy and ileorectal anastomosis. The surgical approach is guided by the findings of the colonic transit study and anorectal manometry study. The results of surgery are variable, and the possible postoperative problems of diarrhoea and faecal incontinence should always be borne in mind.

The results of surgery for outlet delay are also variable. Rectocoele repair, division of the puborectalis for anismus, sphincteroplasty or rectopexy or rectal prolapse are options.

Further reading

Heaton KW, Radvan J, Cripps H *et al*. Defecation frequency and timing, and stool form in the general population. A prospective study. *Gut*, 1992; **33:** 818–24.

McFarlane XA, Morris AI. Faecal incontinence and constipation. *Journal of the Royal College of Physicians of London*, 1997; **31:** 487–92.

Wald A. Colonic and anorectal motility testing in clinical practice. *American Journal of Gastroenterology*, 1994; **89:** 2109–15.

Related topic of interest

Irritable bowel syndrome (p. 176)

CROHN'S DISEASE – BACKGROUND AND CLINICAL FEATURES

Crohn's disease is a chronic transmural granulomatous inflammation which may affect any part of the gastrointestinal tract from the mouth to the anus. Anatomical distribution is as follows (approximate frequency in brackets): ileocaecal (40%), colonic (25%), small bowel only (25%), extensive small bowel (5%), miscellaneous (e.g. confined to ano-rectum, stomach or mouth) (2%).

Incidence and aetiology

In contrast to ulcerative colitis, the incidence of Crohn's disease is increasing. The aetiology remains obscure. One proposal is that, with improved hygiene/medical interventions, fewer children are dying from neonatal enteric infections, and Crohn's disease is a late presentation of persistent infection.

Genetic and environmental factors are involved. The risk of a sibling or parent of a patient developing Crohn's disease is 3–8% (cf. 1–3% in ulcerative colitis). The risk of a patient's child developing Crohn's disease is 1–2% (about the same as for ulcerative colitis). Monozygotic twins are concordant in approximately 50% of cases (more than for ulcerative colitis).

Other aetiological factors proposed are:

- Infective agents (particularly *Mycobacterium paratuberculosis* and childhood-acquired measles).
- A diet high in refined sugar.
- Psychological stress.
- Deranged intestinal cell-mediated immunity.
- HLA subtypes.

Crohn's disease usually presents in the second or third decades, with a smaller peak in the seventh and eighth decades. It is predominantly found in the USA, Northern Europe and Australia where it affects between 30–50 per 100 000 population, irrespective of social class or race. It is commoner in smokers than in non-smokers, in urban areas than in rural areas, and in those on the oral contraceptive pill.

Clinical features

Diarrhoea, abdominal pain, and weight loss are the most common symptoms.

1. Diarrhoea. This may be secondary to many factors:

- Diminished water absorption due to colonic involvement.
- Bacterial overgrowth (due to obstructive stricture, blind loop or fistula formation).
- Impaired bile acid absorption in the terminal ileum (due to disease or surgical resection).
- Proctitis (results in impaired sphincter function and frequent passage of watery stools with mucus).

- Rectal stenosis (causing constipation with overflow diarrhoea).
- Steatorrhoea may occur when >100 cm of the terminal ileum is involved or surgically removed.

2. Abdominal pain. This is often colicky and located in the right-lower quadrant or suprapubic region. Pain may be due to stricturing (in chronic disease), inflammation and spasm (during an acute exacerbation), or a combination of both. Some patients present with acute right iliac fossa pain, tenderness and mass, suggestive of acute appendicitis.

3. Weight loss. This may occur in the absence of other symptoms and may be confused with anorexia nervosa in adolescents. It is usually due to anorexia, diarrhoea, or rarely frank malabsorption (which only occurs in the setting of extensive small-bowel disease).

4. Frank rectal bleeding. This is much less common than in colitis, but will occur in about 40% of those with colonic disease.

5. Peri-anal disease. This includes recurrent abscesses, fissures, fistulae and violaceous skin tags, affects up to 25% of patients, and in some may be the presenting (and only) feature.

6. Other features. These are low-grade fever and malaise, anaemia (due to chronic disease, iron deficiency from chronic blood loss, or rarely malabsorption of vitamin B_{12} and folate) and oral ulceration.

After initial presentation, the disease may evolve into a fibrostenotic or fistulating pattern. The former leads to stricture formation with symptoms of postprandial abdominal pain and constipation; the latter to formation of penetrating sinuses, which may cause intra-abdominal abscesses or fistulae. Fistulae can form between adjacent loops of bowel (entero-enteric); or between bowel and stomach (enterogastric), duodenum (colo-duodenal), bladder (enterovesical), vagina (enterovaginal) or skin (enterocutaneous) – the latter almost invariably in the context of a postoperative complication.

Extra-intestinal manifestations

Extra-intestinal manifestations occur in about 15% of patients and can be divided into three categories.

1. Related to disease (usually predominantly colonic) activity
- Oral disease – stomatitis and aphthous ulceration.
- Skin lesions – erythema nodosum (which may also be due to the sulphapyridine in sulphasalazine) and pyoderma gangrenosum (less common than in ulcerative colitis).

- Ocular manifestations – conjunctivitis, episcleritis, iritis.
- Musculoskeletal manifestations – clubbing, large and small joint oligoarthritis (excluding sacroiliitis which is unrelated to disease activity).
- Hypercoagulability, usually presenting as lower limb thrombosis (often following surgery) or less commonly as ischaemic stroke. Treatment may be problematic due to the exacerbation of gastrointestinal blood loss with anti-coagulants.

2. Malabsorption-related. Malabsorption may result from the short bowel syndrome following surgical resection(s) (the commonest cause), bacterial overgrowth (due to stasis above a stricture, fistulae or a blind loop) or diffuse small bowel disease. The following extra-intestinal problems may result:

- Nutritional deficiencies – fat-soluble vitamins (vitamins A, D, E and K), folate, vitamin B_{12}, iron, calcium, magnesium (which is needed for vitamin D absorption) and trace elements (e.g. selenium, zinc).
- Gallstones due to alterations in the bile-salt pool secondary to ileal disease (15–35% of those with ileal disease develop gallstones).
- Renal stones. Small bowel disease may lead to fat malabsorption. Increased levels of fatty acids in the colon impair oxalate binding, leading to increased systemic absorption and calcium oxalate renal stones. Urate stones are usually seen in those who have had a colectomy.

3. Miscellaneous
- Liver disease – fatty liver due to chronic malnutrition or total parenteral nutrition; PSC complicated by the late development of cholangiocarcinoma (less common than in ulcerative colitis).
- Amyloidosis is a rare complication of long-standing disease which affects multiple organs and usually presents as the nephrotic syndrome.
- Renal disease – oxalate or amyloid nephropathy; 5-ASA-related nephritis; prerenal uraemia due to dehydration; right hydronephrosis.
- Musculoskeletal – sacroiliitis; ankylosing spondylitis (rare); pelvic osteomyelitis due to small bowel fistulae.
- Adverse effects of medication. Some examples include corticosteroids (see below), azathioprine (e.g. macrocytosis, pancreatitis), sulphasalazine (e.g. lymphopenia, folate deficiency).

Investigations

1. Diagnostic investigations

- Barium studies are used to evaluate the extent and severity of disease. Barium follow-through enteroclysis is used to show the extent of disease in the small bowel. Features include:

    Thickened, separated loops of oedematous bowel.

    Mucosal ulceration – aphthoid, 'rose-thorn' or linear ulcers.

    Fissuring with intervening normal mucosa ('skip lesions').

    'Cobblestone' pattern – transverse and longitudinal ulceration separating oedematous areas of mucosa.

    Thickening of valvulae conniventes.

    Stricture.

    Fistulae.

    A barium enema will complement colonoscopy and, in addition, show fistulous tracts and terminal ileum changes.

- Colonoscopy/sigmoidoscopy should be performed and biopsies taken from abnormal areas seen on barium enema (e.g. strictures, filling defects), rectum (to show rectal sparing) and normal mucosa (15% will have microscopic granulomas).
- An abdominal CT scan may be useful in assessing extra-intestinal complications (e.g. fistulous tracts and abscesses).

2. Assessment of disease activity. Disease activity indices combine a number of clinical and laboratory variables; several exist (e.g. Crohn's Disease Activity Index, Oxford Index) but they are impractical for everyday clinical use. No one test of disease activity is sufficiently accurate alone, and the following should be seen as complementary.

- Laboratory tests suggesting disease activity:

    Anaemia.

    Thrombocytosis.

    Leucocytosis.

    Low serum albumin.

    Elevated CRP (one of the most sensitive tests) and ESR (most useful for Crohn's colitis).

- Colonoscopy gives a guide to activity; however, as the disease is transmural macroscopic appearances may correlate poorly with true disease activity.
- [111]In or [99]technetium-HMPAO-labelled leucocyte scanning is useful in localizing the site and extent of inflammation and differentiating inflammatory from fibrotic strictures.

| | • Barium studies are better at assessing disease extent than activity; if previous studies are available the sequential changes (or lack of them) can be useful. |

Differential diagnosis

1. *Other inflammatory diseases*
   - Ulcerative colitis.
   - Radiation colitis.
   - Ischaemic colitis.
   - Systemic vasculitis, including Behçet's disease (characterized by deep mucosal ulceration and orogenital ulcers).

2. *Infections*
   - Tuberculosis (an important differential diagnosis in terminal ileal disease).
   - Bacterial enteritis.
   - Parasitic infection (amoebiasis or schistosomiasis).

3. *Neoplasia*
   - Small bowel lymphoma.
   - Adenocarcinoma.

4. *Conditions producing right-lower quadrant pain/mass*
   - Appendicitis/appendix abscess.
   - Caecal malignancies.
   - Tuberculosis.
   - Amoeboma.
   - Actinomycosis.
   - *Yersinia enterocolitica.*

5. *Gynaecological conditions*
   - Pelvic inflammatory disease.
   - Ovarian cysts.
   - Ectopic pregnancy.
   - Endometriosis.

6. *Other causes of peri-anal disease*
   - Solitary rectal ulcer disease.
   - Carcinoma.
   - Lymphogranuloma venereum.
   - Herpes simplex.
   - Syphilis.
   - Behçet's disease.

Further reading

British Society of Gastroenterology. Inflammatory Bowel Disease. *BSG Guidelines in Gastroenterology*, September 1996.

Forbes A. *Clinicians' Guide to Inflammatory Bowel Disease*. London: Chapman and Hall Medical, 1997.

Hanauer SB. Inflammatory bowel disease. *New England Journal of Medicine*, 1996; **334**: 841–8.

Rhodes JM. Crohn's disease. *Prescribers' Journal*, 1997; **37(4)**: 232–42.

Related topics of interest

CROHN'S DISEASE – MEDICAL AND SURGICAL MANAGEMENT

Medical treatment

This should be considered in two phases: first, treatment of the acute attack to induce remission in new/relapsed disease, and second, the maintenance of remission.

Inducing remission

1. Sulphasalazine and 5-ASA preparations. These are used in mild to moderate disease, particularly when the colon is involved. The therapeutic effect may take 8–12 weeks, and so steroids in some form are often needed for adequate initial symptom control. The different formulations and adverse effects of 5-ASA are outlined in 'Ulcerative colitis – medical and surgical management' (p. 265). Preparations which release in the more proximal bowel (e.g. Pentasa) should have more benefit where the small bowel is affected.

2. Corticosteroids. These are most effective (70–80% will respond). Different preparations include enemas and suppositories, oral prednisolone, oral budesonide and i.v. hydrocortisone. Adverse effects of short courses of corticosteroids include weight gain, acne, mood changes and, rarely, hypertension and hyperglycaemia. Long-term use is associated with an increased risk of osteoporosis (bone densitometry monitoring is needed), avascular bone necrosis (e.g. femoral head) and growth retardation in children.

'Enterocort' (pH-sensitive coated budesonide) is a new steroid released predominantly in the ileocaecal region. It has fewer systemic side-effects than conventional steroids due to a first-pass metabolism of up to 90%. It should be considered for patients with ileocolonic disease and in whom the adverse reactions to corticosteroids need to be avoided.

3. Specialized nutritional therapies. These are as effective as steroids in inducing short-term remission, but are less convenient and more expensive; they may be the first-choice therapy for those with extensive disease or multiple resections of small bowel. They are best suited for motivated adults/children, where avoidance of steroid side-effects is a major benefit.

- Elemental diets contain nutrients in easily assimilable forms (i.e. free amino acids, monosaccharides and small quantities of short-chain triglycerides) and are usually administered via a fine-bore nasogastric tube as they are unpalatable.

- Polymeric preparations contain nitrogen as whole protein and are available in carton form (chilling improves the palatability). They are usually administered instead of steroids for 2–4 weeks, and other oral intake (except water) is avoided. The main adverse effects are nausea and postural hypotension. Those preparations with a very low content of long-chain fat tend to have the best therapeutic response.
- Total parenteral nutrition (TPN) may be used to maintain nutrition in severe cases, possibly prior to surgery; however, it is no better than elemental or polymeric diets in inducing remission.

4. Antibiotics (metronidazole or ciprofloxacin). These are used to treat infective complications in the colon and peri-anal region (e.g. fistulae, bacterial overgrowth and abscesses). Metronidazole may have an effect in the primary treatment of perianal/colonic Crohn's disease (possibly through effects on cell-mediated immunity, free-radical scavenging and granuloma formation). However, nausea is a common side-effect with metronidazole, and prolonged use of >10 mg/kg/day is associated with the risk of peripheral neuropathy.

5. Immunomodulators. Immunomodulators such as azathioprine (2–2.5 mg/kg/day) will induce remission in active Crohn's disease. It is usually not practical as sole therapy as it may take several months to produce a response. Lymphocytopenia occurs in most adequately treated patients. Bone marrow suppression (particularly neutropenia) is the most common serious adverse effect and is usually dose-related. Other side-effects include hypersensitivity reactions, deranged liver enzymes and pancreatitis (3% of patients). Macrocytosis is common and unimportant. Patients should be advised to stop the drug if symptoms of intercurrent infection develop, and full blood counts should be monitored monthly and liver enzymes 6-monthly.

Methotrexate has both immunosuppressant and anti-inflammatory activity and is being increasingly used in active disease. Most studies have shown cyclosporin to be ineffective. A number of other immunomodulators (e.g. tacrolimus (FK506), and antagonists of interleukin-1, interleukin-2 and tumour necrosis factor α) show promise and are currently under review.

Management outline – induction of remission

1. Mild disease
- Out-patient treatment is possible. Treatment without steroids may be possible.

- For predominantly ileal disease, give Pentasa (2–4 g in divided doses). Ileocolonic disease is best treated with Pentasa, or Asacol (2.4–4.8 g in divided doses). Sulphasalazine is useful only for colonic disease.
- Oral metronidazole (400 mg three times a day) or ciprofloxacin is effective for suppurating perianal disease.

2. *Moderate disease.* Treatment is as above, with:
- Prednisolone (30–60 mg per day initially) will induce remission in one-third and considerably improve symptoms in one-third. There are few controlled studies to provide definitive guidelines over dose, duration and rate of reduction. A reasonable approach is to use high doses until symptoms begin to improve, and then to reduce the dose very gradually over 4–6 weeks. For those who relapse, the high-dose course can be re-initiated, and steroids lowered more slowly next time with the addition of a higher dose of 5-ASA preparation and/or azathioprine as additional therapies. For those at risk of side-effects of steroids, budesonide (9 mg daily for up to 8 weeks, thereafter reducing over the next 4–8 weeks) is appropriate.

3. *Severe disease*
- In-patient treatment is necessary, co-ordinated between medical and surgical teams.
- Intravenous replacement of fluid, electrolytes (especially potassium) and blood should be commenced according to the clinical and laboratory findings.
- Oral fluids are permissible. Food may worsen symptoms, and is usually avoided initially.
- Intravenous hydrocortisone (100 mg four times daily) is given initially, and changed to oral prednisolone (40 mg per day) when tolerated. Prednisolone should be gradually reduced over the next 8 weeks. Some patients are very sensitive to minor fluctuations in the dosage and may relapse if the steroids are reduced too rapidly. The aim should always be to stop the steroids completely, as they have no benefit in the long-term prevention of relapse once remission is established.
- Specialized nutritional therapy (see above) should be considered for motivated adults and children. TPN may be required, especially prior to surgery.
- Intravenous metronidazole, changed to oral when tolerated, may be useful in some patients.
- Response should be monitored by symptoms (bowel frequency, anorexia), signs (temperature, abdominal tenderness, bowel sounds) and laboratory tests (full blood count, electrolytes, ESR, CRP, albumin).

Maintenance of remission

In spite of maintenance treatment, approximately 10% of patients relapse each year.

1. 5-ASA compounds. These are less effective in Crohn's disease than in ulcerative colitis (reduce relapse rate by one-third). They are more effective in those with predominantly colonic disease: those with predominant small bowel disease should be given Pentasa.

2. Corticosteroids. These are no more effective in long-term studies (i.e. after about 9 months) at maintaining remission than placebo. Some patients, however, have continuously active disease, and are very sensitive to minor reductions in steroid dose. The lowest possible steroid dose should be used: optimal use of 5-ASA compounds and/or azathioprine can reduce/remove steroid dependence.

3. Azathioprine (1.5–2 mg/kg/day). This is useful as a steroid-sparing agent and is effective in preventing relapse in approximately 70% of patients with chronically active disease. It may enable reduction or withdrawal of steroid therapy in steroid-dependent patients.

4. Stopping smoking and dietary advice. These are important. Vitamin B_{12} may be needed for those with ileal disease. Those with strictures may benefit from a low natural fibre diet with folate and vitamin C supplementation. Some patients have hypolactasia and benefit from withdrawal of dairy products. Systematic elimination of various other foodstuffs may be useful to detect food intolerances.

Specific management problems

1. Mouth ulcers. Hydrocortisone lozenges with or without antiseptic mouthwashes are usually effective. Resistant ulcers should be treated with oral prednisolone, with or without azathioprine.

2. Persistent diarrhoea. Diarrhoea occurring after distal ileal resection or disease may be due to bile-salt malabsorption and may respond to the anion-exchange resin cholestyramine (4 g before each main meal).

Small bowel bacterial overgrowth may occur after ileo-colonic resection or fistula formation. Confirmatory tests and treatment are outlined in 'Malabsorption' (p. 189). If no cause can be found, stool frequency can be reduced with loperamide (2 mg after each loose stool) or codeine phosphate.

A high-output ileostomy may lead to significant dehydration, and if patients respond to the resultant thirst with water or low osmolarity drinks, electrolyte and volume loss is worsened. Expert nutritional input is required, but a simple rule of thumb is that all oral fluids should be at least iso-osmolar (e.g. using World Health Organization (WHO) rehydration solution).

3. Peri-anal disease. Surgical treatment should be reserved for drainage of abscesses and treatment of fistulae unresponsive to medical treatment.

Surgical treatment

Eighty to ninety percent of patients with ileocolonic disease, and approximately 40% of those with colonic disease, require surgery at some stage of their illness. In general, surgery is reserved for complications, or for localized disease unresponsive to medical management.

Specific indications for surgery are:

- Obstruction due to strictures.
- Localized disease, symptomatic despite medical treatment.
- Abscesses which cannot be drained percutaneously.
- Enterocutaneous fistulae.
- Peri-anal infection requiring drainage.
- (Rarely) perforation, bleeding or carcinoma.

Principles of surgery
- Ideally, resection is limited as far as is possible, with a primary anastomosis.
- Recurrence is halved with a stoma compared to an anastomosis.
- Young patients, with disease limited to the ileocaecal region, often do well with a limited resection; however, histological recurrence occurs in the majority. Multiple small intestinal strictures are best treated with strictureoplasty to reduce the risk of short bowel syndrome.
- Severe peri-anal or colonic disease sometimes requires a diverting ileostomy, which is permanent in 75%.

Cancer risk

The overall risk of developing cancer in Crohn's disease is small; patients with complicated anorectal disease are at most risk and should be kept under review. The risk of colon cancer with long-standing colonic disease is increased (probably slightly less so than in ulcerative colitis), as is the risk of adenocarcinoma of the small bowel in long-standing small bowel disease. The degree of increased risk of cancer in Crohn's disease remains controversial, and no screening strategy has been agreed upon.

Useful addresses

National Association for Colitis and Crohn's Disease (NACC)
PO Box 205
St Albans
AL1 1AB
Tel: 01727-844296

British Colostomy Association
15 Station Road
Reading
Berkshire
RG1 1LG

Further reading

British Society of Gastroenterology. Inflammatory Bowel Disease. *BSG Guidelines in Gastroenterology*, September 1996.

Forbes A. *Clinicians' Guide to Inflammatory Bowel Disease*. London: Chapman and Hall Medical, 1997.

Hanauer SB. Inflammatory bowel disease. *New England Journal of Medicine*, 1996; **334**: 841–8.

Rhodes JM. Crohn's disease. *Prescribers' Journal*, 1997; **37(4)**: 232–42.

Related topics of interest

Colitis – non-specific (p. 50)
Crohn's disease – background and clinical features (p. 67)
Diarrhoea (p. 81)
Malabsorption (p. 189)
Ulcerative colitis – background and clinical features (p. 265)
Ulcerative colitis – medical and surgical management (p. 269)

DIABETIC GASTROPARESIS

Impaired gastric motility occurs in 20–30% of all diabetics (insulin-dependent and non-insulin-dependent); however, only a minority are symptomatic. It occurs due to dysfunction of the parasympathetic supply to the stomach via the vagus nerve, and reflects widespread autonomic system disease, usually in long-standing diabetics.

Clinical features Symptoms range from mild abdominal bloating following a meal to nausea and intractable vomiting. Diabetic control worsens with such upper gastrointestinal disturbance, which further aggravates delayed gastric emptying.

Investigations The diagnosis is suspected from the history. A barium meal will reveal a dilated stomach with food residue and a delayed emptying time. If necessary, radiolabelled scintigraphy will confirm the diagnosis. An endoscopy should always be performed to exclude mechanical causes of outflow obstruction such as pyloric stenosis or an antral tumour. Cardiovascular autonomic function tests should be performed, and will invariably be abnormal.

Treatment *1. General measures.* Adequate relief of symptoms is often difficult to attain. Small, frequent meals of low fat and low fibre are advisable. Hypothyroidism should be excluded. Improvement in blood glucose levels may accelerate gastric emptying, and agents that delay emptying (such as tricyclic antidepressants, opiates, phenothiazines and anticholinergics) should be avoided. Chronic renal failure exacerbates gastric autonomic dysfunction and, if possible, this should be corrected.

2. Medical therapy
- Medical therapy with prokinetic agents is often useful. Metoclopramide (10 mg three times a day), domperidone (10–40 mg three times a day) or cisapride (10 mg three times a day) before meals are often effective. Metoclopramide and domperidone may be given intravenously in severe cases. Erythromycin (250 mg three times a day, orally or intravenously) may help.
- Maintaining adequate nutrition is important in severe cases, and this may be achieved temporarily via a nasojejunal tube. For patients requiring long-term feeding, percutaneous feeding tubes can be placed directly into the small bowel endoscopically (if a push-enteroscope is available) or surgically; alternatively, tubes may be passed into the upper small bowel via the stomach through a gastrostomy. Patients are not necessarily confined to such feeding methods for life, as gastroparesis may improve with time.

- Total parenteral nutrition and surgical procedures (pyloroplasty, gastrectomy or gastric jejunostomy) are justified only as a last resort.

Further reading

Dowling CJ, Kumar S, Boulton JM *et al*. Severe gastroparesis diabeticorum in a young patient with insulin-dependent diabetes. *British Medical Journal*, 1995; **310:** 308–11.

Mearin F, Malagelada JR. Gastroparesis and dyspepsia in patients with diabetes mellitus. *European Journal of Gastroenterology and Hepatology*, 1995; **7:** 717–23.

Related topic of interest

Nausea and vomiting (p. 203)

DIARRHOEA

Diarrhoea can be defined as an increase in frequency and liquidity of stools. This is usually accompanied by a daily stool weight of >200 g or a daily volume of >200 ml. The following mechanisms of diarrhoea are recognized.

Osmotic diarrhoea

This is due to unabsorbed osmotically active substances which retain water in the gut lumen. Osmotic diarrhoea characteristically settles with fasting. It is characterized by the presence of a faecal fluid osmotic gap which is calculated as:

Measured stool osmolality (normally about that of plasma, i.e. 290 mOsmol/kg) $-$ 2 $\times$ (stool sodium + stool potassium).

If the osmotic gap is >50 mOsmol/kg, it is worth measuring stool magnesium (normal being <45 mmol/l or 30 meq/day) as a pointer to laxative abuse. Other causes include carbohydrate malabsorption (e.g. generalized malabsorption syndromes, disaccharidase deficiency, lactase deficiency), excessive ingestion of poorly absorbed carbohydrate or other osmotically active substances (e.g. fruit, artificial sweeteners, laxatives).

Secretory diarrhoea

This is characterized by the absence of an osmotic gap, and the persistence of symptoms (usually a large stool volume of >400 ml/day) with fasting. The diarrhoea results from a reduced ion and water absorption or the secretion of ions and water into the gut lumen. This arises either due to diffuse mucosal disease (e.g. inflammatory bowel disease, lymphoma, coeliac disease, tropical sprue, collagen vascular diseases), intestinal resection (which causes bile salt malabsorption) or abnormal mediators acting on intracellular cyclic adenosine monophosphate (cAMP), calcium and protein kinases. Such abnormal mediators include neurohormonal agents (e.g. carcinoid syndrome, Zollinger–Ellison syndrome, vipoma, hyperthyroidism), bacterial enterotoxins (e.g. enterotoxigenic *Escherichia coli*, *Vibrio cholerae*, *Staphylococcus aureus*, *Clostridium perfringens*), stimulant laxatives (e.g. senna, bisacodyl, phenolphthalein) and bile acids.

Abnormal motility

Deranged intestinal motility is difficult to confirm and the diagnosis is usually made after excluding osmotic and secretory causes. Possible examples of increased motility are the irritable bowel syndrome, postgastrectomy, diabetic gastropathy, carcinoid syndrome, hyperthyroidism and drugs (e.g. stimulant laxatives, prokinetics, erythromycin).

Combined mechanisms

In many cases the cause of diarrhoea is multifactorial. Examples include acute infectious diarrhoea (direct toxin-induced effects and abnormal motility) and ulcerative colitis (altered mucosal permeability and absorption as epithelial cells are inflamed, prostaglandin and short-chain fatty acid-induced mucosal damage, deranged motility, decreased rectal capacity and exudation of blood and mucus into the lumen).

Clinical evaluation

1. *History.* Enquire about recent travel, contacts, drugs (laxatives, antibiotics, immunosuppressant treatment, over-the-counter remedies, herbal preparations), alcohol intake, sexual history, family history (inflammatory bowel disease, colon cancer, CD, multiple endocrine neoplasia syndromes), risk factors for HIV, arthritis (inflammatory bowel disease, Whipple's disease, *Yersinia* enteritis, connective tissue disease), frequent infections (hypogammaglobulinaemia, AIDS).

2. *Character of stools*
- Large-volume stools, light in colour, watery or greasy, often containing undigested food particles and no blood, and associated with colicky pain, are likely to be due to disease of the small bowel or proximal colon.
- Frequent, small-volume stools, often with blood or mucus and tenesmus, are likely to be caused by disease in the colon or rectum.
- Diarrhoea (often in the mornings) alternating with constipation, often with the passage of mucus, is suggestive of the irritable bowel syndrome (although a carcinoma of the colon should be excluded in those >45 years old).
- Nocturnal diarrhoea, weight loss or bloody diarrhoea all suggest an organic cause.

3. *Examination*
(a) General examination
- Dehydration.
- Anaemia.
- Skin lesions (erythema nodosum, hyperpigmentation, dermatitis herpetiformis, purpura).
- Clubbing (in some cases of Crohn's disease).
- Goitre (thyrotoxicosis).
- Lymphadenopathy.
(b) Abdominal examination
- Previous operations.
- Hepatosplenomegaly.
- Masses (a right iliac fossa mass could be due to a caecal carcinoma, Crohn's disease, lymphoma, tuberculosis, yersiniosis or an amoeboma).

- A rectal examination is mandatory to detect tumours or faecal impaction.

Investigations

Diarrhoea should be investigated if it persists for longer than 3 weeks, or is associated with weight loss or dehydration. The following tests should be tailored according to the information gained from the history and examination.

1. *Blood tests.* Screening blood tests should include:

- Full blood count, erythrocyte sedimentation rate (ESR) and C-reactive protein (CRP) (which are raised, sometimes independently, and not invariably, in inflammatory bowel disease, carcinoma and infections).
- Electrolytes (hypokalaemia can occur in prolonged diarrhoea due to laxative abuse, rectal villous adenoma or a vipoma).
- Albumin (low in protein-losing enteropathy, most inflammatory conditions and most malabsorption states).
- Immunoglobulins (low in hypogammaglobulinaemia).
- Thyroid function tests.
- Anti-gliadin antibodies (particularly if there is evidence of iron deficiency).
- Red cell folate and vitamin B_{12}.

2. *Sigmoidoscopy and colonoscopy.* A rigid sigmoidoscopy is usually performed initially and does not require prior bowel preparation. This allows direct visualization of the mucosa and biopsies to be taken (ulcerative colitis, Crohn's disease, pseudomembranous colitis and amoebic ulcers are possible findings). A colonoscopy (to the terminal ileum) is usually necessary if the rigid sigmoidoscopy is inconclusive. It is important to biopsy each part of the colon, as the mucosa may appear macroscopically normal in certain diseases (e.g. Crohn's disease, microscopic or collagenous colitis).

3. *Oesophagogastroduodenoscopy.* A biopsy should be taken from the second part of the duodenum (or the jejunum if an enteroscope is available) to detect CD, lymphoma, Crohn's disease, Whipple's disease, lymphangiectasia or giardiasis). A jejunal aspiration and culture may be performed if small-bowel bacterial overgrowth and giardiasis is considered.

4. *Stool specimen.* A random fresh stool specimen should be obtained and analysed for the presence of blood, leucocytes, cysts (especially *Cryptosporidium* if immunocompromised), parasites (particularly *Giardia lamblia* trophozoites), ova and bacteria. The stool may be cultured for *Salmonella, Shigella, Campylobacter* and *Yersinia* spp. Toxin assays may be performed for *Clostridium difficile* toxin and *E. coli* toxin. Other

tests include a Sudan stain for fat, pH analysis, anionic gap, occult blood test and alkalinization for phenolphthalein.

5. Barium enema. This is useful to assess the extent and complications of inflammatory bowel disease.

6. Small-bowel barium studies. Small-bowel barium follow-through may show features of Crohn's disease, jejunal diverticulosis, small-bowel lymphoma, abdominal tuberculosis or systemic sclerosis.

7. CT scan of the abdomen. The presence of retroperitoneal tumours (e.g. pancreatic carcinoma), intra-abdominal lymphadenopathy and Crohn's disease will be revealed.

8. Endoscopic retrograde cholangiopancreatography. An ERCP, with the necessary pancreatic malabsorption tests, will confirm suspected chronic pancreatitis.

In-patient investigations

In most cases, the above investigations will reveal the diagnosis. For a small number of patients, in-patient assessment is needed. The response to 3 days of fasting and the collection of a 3-day faecal specimen for weight, fat and osmolality is valuable. A stool weight of <200 g/day (on a normal diet) is unlikely to be pathological and suggests a functional bowel disorder. Patients passing more than this should collect a 24-hour urine specimen for 5-hydroxyindoleacetic acid (5-HIAA) levels (to detect possible carcinoid syndrome), have blood taken for gastrin, vasoactive intestinal peptide (VIP) and calcitonin levels and have a bile-acid breath test performed.

Those patients found to have osmotic diarrhoea require tests for carbohydrate malabsorption (i.e. a lactose breath test (to detect lactase deficiency) or lactulose breath test (to detect small-bowel bacterial overgrowth)). Laxative abuse can be excluded with stool and urine laxative assays.

General principles for treatment of diarrhoea

- Rehydration therapy and correction of malnutrition is more important than establishing a cause in severe cases.
- Ideally the cause should be found and treated before symptomatic treatment is given.
- Stool frequency can usually be controlled with either titrated doses of codeine phosphate or loperamide, and occasionally both. These are contraindicated in children (due to the risk of paralytic ileus) and in severe colitis of any cause (toxic dilatation is a risk). They should be avoided in infectious diarrhoea if possible (due to a theoretical risk of delayed clearance of the organism and a probable increased risk of infectious complications).

- Only confirmed infectious diarrhoea due to *Giardia lamblia*, *Yersinia enterocolitica*, *Salmonella typhi*, *E. coli* and *Campylobacter jejuni* and shigellosis should be treated with antibiotics. Antibiotic treatment of non-typhoidal salmonellosis should be avoided as this prolongs the excretion of the organism and increases the risk of a carrier state.
- The treatment of the malabsorption syndromes and the irritable bowel syndrome are covered in the appropriate chapters.

Further reading

Turnberg LA. Pathophysiology of diarrhoea. In: Misicwicz JJ, Pounder RE, Venables CW (eds). *Diseases of the Gut and Pancreas*. Oxford: Blackwell Scientific Ltd, 1994; 37–50.

Related topics of interest

Malabsorption (p. 189)
Irritable bowel syndrome (p. 176)

DUODENAL ULCERS

Duodenal ulcers (DU) are more common in men, and are three times as common as gastric ulcers in patients below the age of 40. Most occur within the first 2 cm of the duodenum, and 95% are associated with *Helicobacter pylori* infection. See also 'Helicobacter pylori' (p. 145).

Aetiology

- Most (90–95%) cases of duodenal ulceration are associated with *H. pylori* infection and acid hypersecretion. However, other host and environmental factors must contribute to the aetiology, as only a minority of those with gastric *H. pylori* infection will develop DU.
- Drugs account for most other cases of DU; steroids (when used with NSAIDs), NSAIDs and aspirin are the main culprits. The elderly and those on long-term therapy and higher doses are at greatest risk.
- Acute gastroduodenal ulcers may develop as a result of severe physiological stress. Curling's ulcers can develop when burns involve greater than 35% of the body's surface area. Cushing's ulcers are those that develop after central nervous system trauma or in the intensive therapy unit (ITU) setting, particularly in those who are comatose or receiving artificial ventilation. They have a high incidence of complications, and are a significant cause of morbidity in ITU patients.

Rare causes

These include the Zollinger–Ellison syndrome (see p. 210), hyperparathyroidism (and possibly other causes of hypercalcaemia), systemic mastocytosis, annular pancreas and herpes simplex virus infection. Those with hepatic cirrhosis or chronic lung disease have an increased incidence of DU.

- Postbulbar ulcers (those occurring beyond 3 cm of the pylorus) are rare, and warrrant investigation for atypical aetiologies (e.g. Crohn's disease, Zollinger–Ellison syndrome, ectopic pancreatic tissue, lymphoma, carcinoma, tuberculosis).

Other factors

- Although spicy foods cause dyspepsia, none have been clearly linked to DU.
- Alcohol causes acute mucosal damage but not DU.
- Psychological factors are known to affect the gastrointestinal and immune systems, but the link with DU disease is difficult to quantify.
- Smoking increases the incidence of duodenal disease in a dose-dependent manner. Smoking also increases the risk of relapse and complications.

Clinical features	No group of symptoms are characteristic, and the severity of symptoms often have no correlation with the severity of disease.

- A relatively common symptom is epigastric pain (often burning or cramping) which occurs between meals (hunger pain) and may variably be relieved by antacids. The pain often occurs in clusters of a few weeks at a time and, like gastric ulcers, may occur at night. Pain radiating to the back suggests a posterior ulcer.
- Elderly patients and those on NSAIDs (50% of cases) may have no symptoms or atypical symptoms ('silent' ulcers). Such patients often present with complications without preceding dyspepsia.
- Physical examination may be normal or reveal epigastric tenderness. Features of pyloric outlet obstruction or perforation may be elicited rarely.

Diagnosis of *H. pylori* infection

The presence of *H. pylori* can be detected serologically, by breath tests, or by endoscopic biopsy (rapid urease test, histology or culture). While most of the tests are accurate, they carry a 5–15% false-negative rate overall. No one test is perfect, and the choice of test depends on the clinical situation.

- Those patients <45 years old with a history of dyspepsia should be tested serologically, and if positive are usually recommended for endoscopic examination. Negative serology in patients not on NSAIDs makes the diagnosis of DU disease very unlikely.
- Older patients with new-onset non-reflux dyspepsia are usually referred for an endoscopy and rapid urease biopsy test (e.g. *Campylobacter*-like organism urease test ('Clotest')). False-positive results are rare with the rapid urease tests. False-negative results can occur with the use of proton pump inhibitors, bismuth or antibiotics, which all temporarily suppress *H. pylori*.
- To confirm eradication after therapy, a ^{13}C or ^{14}C breath test should be used.

Other investigations

- Routine biopsy of duodenal ulcers is not needed, unless unusual causes are suspected (see above).
- A full blood count may reveal anaemia if bleeding has occurred.
- If ulceration is atypical in location or rapidly recurrent, or a significant family history is elicited, serum calcium and fasting gastrin should be checked (after stopping acid-suppressing drugs).

Management – general measures

- Stopping smoking improves healing and decreases the rate of relapse.

- Alcohol intake above the recommended 14 units per week for women and 21 units per week for men should be avoided.
- NSAIDs and aspirin should be avoided if possible.

**Management –
medical treatment**

1. H. pylori eradication

- *H. pylori* eradication can effect primary ulcer healing, decreases ulcer recurrence and reduces the risk of recurrent complications.
- Various combinations of an antisecretory agent together with two antibiotics exist; however, the optimal frequency, dose and duration of treatment has not been determined.
- A realistic eradication treatment regimen is one of a week's duration with a cure rate of at least 90%. One such regimen is omeprazole (20 mg twice daily before meals), metronidazole (400 mg twice daily with meals) and clarithromycin (500 mg twice daily with meals).
- Three problems limit the effectiveness of regimens to eradicate *H. pylori*:
  - (a) Metronidazole and clarithromycin resistance, usually in those who have received these drugs as monotherapy before. For such patients, metronidazole or clarithromycin may be replaced with amoxicillin (1 g twice daily with meals).
  - (b) Minor adverse reactions occur in 30–50% of patients and include nausea, diarrhoea, allergic reactions to amoxicillin, and a metallic taste with metronidazole and clarithromycin.
  - (c) Patient compliance is often poor due to complicated regimens and adverse effects.
- Successful eradication should be confirmed with a ^{13}C breath test. False negatives occur in up to 10% of cases, especially in the first 3 months after eradication therapy. Errors can be minimized by strict protocols: avoid proton pump inhibitors for 4 weeks prior to testing, antibiotics for 2 weeks and H_2 receptor antagonists for 3 days.
- Recurrence of peptic ulcers is usually due to unsuccessful eradication of *H. pylori*.
- Once cure has been achieved, reinfection has been shown to occur at a rate of <0.5% per annum.

2. Conventional ulcer healing therapy

- This is used in most patients, regardless of *H. pylori* status, to facilitate healing and to relieve symptoms.
- H_2 receptor antagonists, proton pump inhibitors and sucralfate are all safe and effective.
- Ranitidine (300 mg at night) has been shown to heal about 90% of ulcers at 6 weeks. Sucralfate has a similar efficacy.

Omeprazole (20–40 mg daily) (or lansoprazole, 30 mg daily) before meals produces a more rapid healing and symptom relief than the H_2 receptor antagonists, but has similar results after 6–8 weeks.

3. *Refractory ulcers*
- If symptoms remain after 4 weeks of therapy, high-dose acid-suppression therapy should be taken for a further 4 weeks.
- Endoscopy should be repeated if symptoms persist after this. If the ulcer has not healed it should be biopsied to exclude unusual causes, such as Crohn's disease or lymphoma. Biopsies for the rapid urease test should be repeated, including one from the body of the stomach (the organism migrates to the body after prolonged acid suppression).
- A high dose of a proton pump inhibitor such as omeprazole 40 mg daily or lansoprazole 30 mg daily should be given for a further 8 weeks. This heals most ulcers resistant to H_2 receptor antagonists.
- Fasting serum gastrin levels should be considered (off acid-suppression therapy). Patient compliance, smoking habit and NSAID or aspirin use should be checked.

4. *Maintenance therapy*
- Persistent *H. pylori* infection is the major determinant for ulcer recurrence. Once this is eradicated, maintenance therapy is generally not needed.
- Maintenance therapy may be considered for those with *H. pylori*-negative ulcers, high-risk patients with a history of complications or frequent relapse (more than one every 6 months), and for those who continue to smoke or take NSAIDs.
- Half strength H_2 receptor antagonists are effective at maintaining remission in most cases. Full-dose maintenance H_2 receptor antagonists may be used for high-risk cases. Proton pump inhibitors are only indicated for maintenance of refractory ulcers, or where NSAID use continues (H_2 receptor antagonists do not heal or prevent the commonly occurring NSAID-induced gastric lesions).
- The duration of maintenance therapy has not been agreed upon; however, for those with continuing risk factors (e.g. resistant *H. pylori* infection or NSAIDs), therapy should probably continue for as long as the risk factor remains.
- The safety of long-term proton pump inhibitor use has been called into question. Preliminary studies suggest that long-term use, particularly in patients with continuing *H.*

pylori infection, might accelerate the effects of chronic gastritis (intestinal metaplasia, atrophy, dysplasia, neoplasia). Prolonged hypochlorhydria might promote gastric bacterial overgrowth, and the effects of prolonged hypergastrinaemia might also be cause for concern; no proof of long-term harm in humans exists, but these theoretical dangers should be borne in mind, particularly when considering long-term proton pump inhibitor therapy in young patients.

5. *Treatment of NSAID-associated DU*
- *H. pylori* should be eradicated if present (although this is contentious), and the dose of NSAID should be reduced or stopped.
- Standard H_2 receptor antagonists and proton pump inhibitors will heal most ulcers.
- A proton pump inhibitor should be used to treat large, complicated ulcers if NSAIDs cannot be discontinued.

6. *Prevention of NSAID ulcers*
- For those patients on NSAIDs, anti-ulcer prophylaxis should be considered in the following settings:
    Prior ulcer disease.
    Co-therapy with steroids or anticoagulants.
    Comorbid conditions which would compromise tolerance to complications.
- Although those over the age of 70 (particularly women) are at an increased risk of NSAID-induced ulceration, age in itself is not an indication for anti-ulcer therapy.
- Misoprostol (a prostaglandin E_1 analogue) has been shown to limit NSAID-induced ulcer complications by about 40% (but mainly gastric events). Diarrhoea and abdominal cramps limit patient compliance, but these are often transient.
- Proton pump inhibitors are suitable alternatives if misoprostol is not tolerated.
- The decision to eradicate incidental *H. pylori* infection in those taking NSAIDs is controversial.

Complications
- Haemorrhage and perforation are becoming less common, possibly as a result of *H. pylori* eradication treatments, and potent acid-suppression drugs.
- Pyloric stenosis is recognizable by postprandial vomiting and the findings of a succussion splash, hypokalaemic alkalosis and dehydration. Endoscopic balloon dilatation and high-dose acid-suppression therapy can avert the need for surgery in certain patients.

Surgical management
- Indications:
  Haemorrhage – not controlled by endoscopic therapy.
  Perforation.
  Pyloric stenosis.
  Frequent relapses, especially following a complication, or in the elderly.
- Highly selective vagotomy is the safest elective operation with the fewest side-effects and metabolic adverse effects. The relapse rate is related to the experience of the surgeon and the technique used. It can be performed laparoscopically in certain centres.
- Vagotomy and pyloroplasty are also performed, but are associated with a higher incidence of side-effects (10–15% have dumping, diarrhoea or vomiting).

Further reading

Peura DA. Proceedings of a symposium. *Helicobacter pylori*: from theory to practice. *American Journal of Medicine*, 1996; **100(5A):** 1S–64S.
Soll AH. Consensus statement. Medical treatment of peptic ulcer disease. Practice guidelines. *Journal of the American Medical Association*, 1996; **275:** 622–9.

Related topics of interest

Dyspepsia (p. 92)
Gastric ulcers (p. 108)
Helicobacter pylori (p. 145)

DYSPEPSIA

Dyspepsia (or indigestion) refers to a wide array of upper gastrointestinal tract symptoms, which may be caused by a large number of disorders. Typical symptoms include abdominal discomfort related to meals (or at certain times of the day), anorexia, vomiting, bloating, belching and heartburn. Dyspepsia is common (approximately 30% of the population are affected; about 5% consult their doctor). The personal and economic burden to patients and health carers is considerable.

Dyspepsia either has an identifiable cause such as a duodenal ulcer (organic dyspepsia), or else investigation shows no relevant organic lesion (non-ulcer dyspepsia).

Aetiology of organic dyspepsia

1. *Gastrointestinal disorders*
- GORD
- Peptic ulcer disease.
- Gastritis.
- Duodenitis.
- Biliary colic.
- Chronic pancreatitis.
- Carcinoma (stomach, pancreas).
- Postsurgical stomach.

2. *Metabolic*
- Diabetic gastroparesis.
- Hypercalcaemia.
- Thyroid disorders.

3. *Drugs*
- NSAIDs.
- Steroids.
- Ethanol.
- Antibiotics (e.g. tetracyclines, macrolides).
- Theophylline.

4. *Miscellaneous*
- Ischaemic heart disease.

The common diagnoses made at endoscopy, in all ages, are shown in *Table 1*.

Table 1. Common causes of organic dyspepsia

Cause	Occurrence (%)
Oesophagitis	10–17
Duodenal ulcer	10–15
Gastric ulcer	5–10
Gastritis, duodenitis	30
Hiatus hernia	20
Gastric cancer	2

Aetiology of 'non-ulcer' dyspepsia

There are two broad possibilities: (i) there *is* a pathophysiological abnormality, but it has either not been picked up by the test (e.g. many patients with pathological GORD have a normal-looking oesophagus), or the correct test has not been done (e.g. ultrasound for gallstones); or (ii) *no* pathological disturbance exists (true functional dyspepsia): symptoms are often attributable to stress or other psychological disturbance. Overall this group accounts for around 50% of patients with dyspepsia.

It is likely that multiple factors lead to dyspeptic symptoms in true non-ulcer dyspepsia. The three most important are:

1. Impaired motor and sensory functions. Many such patients have impaired gastric emptying, but there is no correlation between the degree of impairment and symptoms. Intestinal dysmotility is also common in more severe cases. Evidence is accumulating that hypersensitivity of visceral afferent pathways may play a role. This may occur at the peripheral mechanoreceptor level, or in higher brain centres.

2. Mucosal inflammation. Chronic gastritis of varying severity is a recognized complication of *H. pylori* infection, chemical irritants (e.g. alcohol, bile) and autoimmune attack. In cases of *H. pylori* infection, without macroscopic mucosal damage (i.e. ulcers/erosions), studies have often failed to show that the infection is relevant to the symptoms. Similarly, there are no clear data for the role of (non-ulcerative) chemical or autoimmune gastritis in the causation of dyspeptic symptoms. There is no uniform agreement at present on how best to advise patients in these situations.

3. Psychosocial factors. It is widely believed (although scientifically unproven) that psychological stress and significant life events are important in the cause of functional dyspepsia. Patients are also more likely to display anxiety, neurotic behaviour and hypochondriasis. However, these traits are also common in those with organic causes of dyspepsia. No specific personality trait has been causally linked to those with functional dyspepsia.

Assessment

Dyspeptic symptoms are very non-discriminatory between the various organic diseases, and between organic and functional dyspepsia. Clinical features that have the best discriminatory power are given below:

- Dysphagia suggests oesophageal disease, and should always be investigated. A carcinoma of the oesophagus or gastric cardia should always be suspected in older patients.
- Patients who complain of a burning or rising retrosternal pain, reflux of acid or gastric contents to the mouth, and relief of these symptoms with antacids are likely to have GORD (approximately 70% positive predictive value).

- Biliary disease is often distinguishable from upper gastrointestinal pathology by the site, nature and radiation of pain, and the intermittence of symptoms (see 'Gallstone disease' (p. 101)).
- 'Alarm signals' suggest an organic cause, e.g. unintentional weight loss, anorexia, iron deficiency anaemia, haematemesis or melaena, dysphagia, previous gastric surgery, persistent vomiting, epigastric mass, previous peptic ulcer, NSAID use, suspicious radiological examination or waking from sleep.

Guidelines for the investigation of dyspepsia

Currently, dyspepsia is investigated according to the patient's age, *H. pylori* status, and the presence or absence of 'warning' signs (as above).

The following advice is based around the current British Society of Gastroenterology guidelines:

- Any patient over the age of 45 with new-onset dyspepsia should undergo an endoscopy. The presence of 'alarm signals' may necessitate an urgent endoscopy.
- Patients with dyspepsia below the age of 45 who have 'warning signs' should undergo an endoscopy.
- Patients with dyspepsia, below the age of 45 and with no 'warning signs' should have a serological test for *H. pylori*. Those who have *H. pylori* antibodies and remain symptomatic after eradication therapy (see 'Helicobacter pylori' (p. 145)) should undergo an endoscopy. Those who have a negative test should be reassured and treated empirically.

An endoscopy is not necessary in the following circumstances:

- 'Routine' follow-up of a patient with a duodenal ulcer.
- Patients under the age of 45 who have remained asymptomatic after a single episode of dyspepsia (those with a positive serological test for *H. pylori* should have an endoscopy if they become symptomatic).
- Patients who have recently undergone a satisfactory endoscopy for the same symptoms.

The rationale for these guidelines takes the following facts into account: less than 3% of stomach cancers present below the age of 45; those that do usually manifest 'alarm signals' or occur in *H. pylori*-positive patients.

Although reflux oesophagitis and Barrett's oesophagus may be missed by these guidelines, treatment for these conditions is currently based on symptom control, rather than healing.

Treatment of functional dyspepsia

Patients less than 45 years old with a negative *H. pylori* serological test should be treated as 'functional dyspepsia'. Failure to respond to such treatment warrants an endoscopy. Patients over 45, with negative investigation results, are treated similarly. Further management is facilitated by addressing the predominant symptom.

- Reflux-like dyspepsia. Symptoms are predominantly those of GORD. Such patients have no objective evidence of GORD, and the symptoms usually do not respond to acid-suppression therapy. The term 'irritable oesophagus' is sometimes used.
- Dysmotility-like dyspepsia. Symptoms of upper abdominal discomfort, postprandial nausea, bloating and early satiety predominate. The irritable bowel syndrome (IBS) often coexists. Intestinal dysmotility and impaired gastric emptying are thought to be important.
- Ulcer-like dyspepsia. Symptoms are of episodic epigastric pain simulating peptic ulcer disease but with no evidence of peptic ulceration. There is little evidence that acid hypersecretion plays a role, and the symptoms respond poorly to acid-suppressant agents.
- Non-specific dyspepsia. Many patients do not fit exactly into any of the above groups, and may have some features of all three.

1. General measures
- Reassurance and explanation is imperative.
- Lifestyle advice
    Stopping smoking.
    Weight reduction.
    Avoiding coffee, chocolates and excessive alcohol.
    Avoiding medication associated with dyspepsia if possible (e.g. theophylline, NSAIDs, etc).
    Eating regular meals.
These often help, but have not been established scientifically.

2. Drug treatment. Scientific evidence for specific treatments is lacking, and treatment is largely empirical.

- Antacids. Controlled studies have not shown them to be superior to placebo; however, they are safe and well tolerated when used on an as-required basis. Magnesium-based compounds (e.g. magnesium hydroxide) tend to have a diarrhoeal effect, and may be used tactically in those with associated constipation. Aluminium-based compounds (e.g. aluminium hydroxide) tend to be constipating and are preferred in those with frequent or loose stools.
- Dysmotility-type dyspepsia. Prokinetic agents (e.g. domperidone, 10–20 mg three times a day, or cisapride, 10 mg three times a day with meals) may be beneficial. Domperidone blocks dopamine receptors, causing increased

motility in the oesophagus, stomach and small bowel. Lower oesophageal sphincter tone is also increased. Cisapride is structurally related to metoclopramide and is thought to act by potentiating acetylcholine release in the upper gastrointestinal tract. It may be beneficial if symptoms are suggestive of impaired gastric emptying. Cisapride may cause diarrhoea and colic, which is often alleviated with a slow introduction. It also has important drug interactions and should be avoided in those with a cardiac history as it may prolong the Q–T interval and precipitate ventricular dysrythmias.

Antispasmodic agents (e.g. mebeverine, 135 mg three times a day) are sometimes useful and act by directly relaxing intestinal smooth muscle.

- Reflux-type dyspepsia. H_2 receptor antagonists (e.g. ranitidine, 150 mg twice daily), proton pump inhibitors (e.g. omeprazole, 20 mg daily), prokinetic agents (e.g. cisapride, 10 mg three times a day) and alginates (e.g. Gaviscon, 10 ml three times a day) may all be useful.
- Ulcer-type dyspepsia. An H_2 receptor antagonists (e.g. ranitidine, 150 mg twice a day) or a proton pump inhibitor (e.g. omeprazole 20 mg daily) should be tried.

Treatment of duodenal ulcer (including erosive duodenitis)

- Ninety-five percent of cases can be shown to be associated with *H. pylori* infection. Some gastroenterologists would treat *all* cases with *H. pylori* eradication therapy.
- There is no ideal eradication regimen, but most centres now prescribe 1 week of triple therapy with a proton pump inhibitor (omeprazole, 20 mg twice daily, or lansoprazole, 30 mg twice daily) plus amoxicillin (1 g twice daily) plus one other antibiotic (metronidazole, 400 mg twice daily, or clarithromycin, 250–500 mg twice daily).
- Ideally, after 4 weeks (during which proton pump inhibitors should not be used), a carbon-13 breath test should be performed to confirm eradication. If the test is positive, an alternative eradication regimen is given, and the breath test repeated.
- Duodenal ulcers associated with NSAID use should receive acid-suppression therapy, and, if possible, NSAIDs should be avoided. Those patients who are unable to stop NSAIDs should receive long-term acid-suppression therapy. Relapse or persistence of symptoms is an indication for a repeat OGD.

Gastric ulcer

- At endoscopy, the ulcer must be biopsied to exclude malignancy, and a direct urease test should be performed, remembering that the current use of a proton pump inhibitor may produce a false-negative result. *H. pylori* infection is present in 70% of benign gastric ulcers.

- Patients with *H. pylori* infection should receive eradication therapy (as above), followed by acid-suppressant therapy for 2 months to assist healing. Patients without *H. pylori* infection should receive a proton pump inhibitor for 2 months. NSAIDs should be discontinued, or, if this is not possible, taken with a proton pump inhibitor or misoprostol.
- A repeat endoscopy and biopsies are essential to confirm healing and the benign nature of the ulcer. Surgery should be considered for benign ulcers that have not healed after 6 months.

Oesophagitis

- *H. pylori* infection is not involved in the pathogenesis, and eradication may even make control of reflux symptoms worse (one reason being that the hypochlorhydric effect of proton pump inhibitors seems enhanced in the presence of *H. pylori* infection).
- Patients should be advised on 'lifestyle modification', i.e. weight reduction, avoiding large infrequent (fatty) meals – especially late at night, propping up the head of the bed, alcohol and caffeine reduction, smoking cessation, and avoiding tight-fitting garments.
- Treatment is aimed at symptom control, and a repeat endoscopy is not needed to confirm healing. A 4-week course of a proton pump inhibitor, with or without cisapride, is usually beneficial.
- Complicated oesophagitis (e.g. peptic stricture, oesophageal ulceration, bleeding or Barrett's oesophagus) may need follow-up endoscopies, depending on the initial findings.

Non-erosive duodenitis and gastritis

Although these are relatively common findings at endoscopy, they correlate poorly with symptoms and the histological findings. Therapy is therefore empirical, and should involve the cheapest agent which is able to control symptoms.

Further reading

British Society of Gastroenterology. Dyspepsia Management Guidelines. *Guidelines in Gastroenterology*, September 1996.

Holtmann G, Talley NJ. Functional dyspepsia: current treatment recommendations. *Drugs*, 1993; **45(6)**: 918–30.

Malagelada JR. Functional dyspepsia. Insights on mechanisms and management strategies. *Gastroenterology Clinics of North America*, 1996; **25(1)**: 103–12.

Related topics of interest

DYSPHAGIA

Dysphagia refers to the sensation of food being held up in its passage to the stomach. Whilst psychiatric disorders and anxiety states may be the explanation (see below), dysphagia should always be investigated. In all cases, obtaining an adequate history cannot be overemphasized. Dysphagia can be classified into two types: oropharyngeal and oesophageal.

Oropharyngeal (transfer) dysphagia describes difficulty initiating swallowing, or problems with the co-ordination of the swallowing reflex. Symptoms include pain, choking, coughing or regurgitation shortly after swallowing. Causes include:

- Neuromuscular disorders (e.g. stroke, motor neurone disease, bulbar palsy, pseudobulbar palsy, Parkinson's disease, syringomyelia, myotonic dystrophy).
- Local diseases in the mouth (e.g. aphthous ulcers, candidiasis, tumours).
- Pharyngeal pouch (Zenker's diverticulum).

Oesophageal dysphagia refers to food sticking after swallowing. A useful approach is to identify whether dysphagia is to (1) only solids initially, progressing to liquids over time in some cases, or (2) both solids and liquids from the onset.

Dysphagia with only solids initially indicates a mechanical obstruction. If this is episodic and occurs only with certain foods (particularly bread or steak), an oesophageal web or distal oesophageal ring (e.g. Schatzki's ring) should be considered. If the dysphagia with solids is progressive and occurs daily, a diagnosis of carcinoma of the oesophagus or cardia should be strongly suspected, especially if it occurs in someone over the age of 50 and is associated with weight loss. Associated reflux symptoms make a benign peptic stricture more likely (about 10% of those with GORD develop benign oesophageal strictures at some stage in their illness). Rare causes of mechanical dysphagia include extrinsic compression (from a bronchial carcinoma, mediastinal lymph nodes, aortic aneurysm, left atrial enlargement or retrosternal goitre), benign oesophageal tumour, and radiation- or caustic-induced strictures.

Those patients with dysphagia initially with both solids and liquids will probably have a motility disorder. If the symptoms are progressing, the diagnosis is likely to be achalasia (especially if regurgitation of undigested food is a symptom) or scleroderma (where other systemic features will be evident). Diffuse oesophageal spasm is a further possibility, and may be associated with atypical retrosternal chest pain.

Odynophagia

This means 'painful swallowing', usually described as a burning or sharp retrosternal chest discomfort occurring after swallowing, especially with hot or alcoholic drinks. This is usually caused by some form of oesophagitis. Causes include:

- Peptic oesophagitis due to GORD.
- Oesophagitis following ingestion of caustic substances.
- Medication-induced oesophagitis (e.g. antibiotics, potassium chloride, quinidine or the bisphosphonates (particularly alendronate)).
- Infections (e.g. cytomegalovirus, herpes simplex virus, *Candida albicans*), particularly in the immunocompromised.

Globus sensation

Globus sensation ('globus hystericus' is an outdated term) refers to the persistent sensation of a lump in the throat which is often relieved by swallowing (thus distinguishing it from a mechanical obstruction). Physiological causes may play a role: manometric studies have shown cricopharyngeal dysmotility in some patients, and psychiatric disorders are frequently found (most commonly anxiety, depression and somatization disorder). Heartburn is a common concomitant feature and some patients find relief of globus symptoms with antireflux treatment.

Assessment and investigations

- Patients with a recent onset of dysphagia require *urgent* investigation. Because of the danger of perforation, e.g. of an oesophageal pouch, many centres advise a barium swallow rather than endoscopy as the first test.
- All patients should be examined for signs of weight loss, pallor, lymphadenopathy (e.g. a supraclavicular node in carcinoma of the stomach) and the presence or absence of dentures or oral disease. Cranial nerve lesions (particularly tongue and palatal abnormalities) and signs of connective tissue diseases should also be sought.
- Blood tests may reveal dehydration or anaemia (due to iron deficiency secondary to bleeding from a carcinoma or associated with a postcricoid web; or nutritional deficiencies).
- A chest radiograph may show a mediastinal mass (bronchial tumour or lymph nodes), absent gastric bubble and mediastinal fluid level (hiatus hernia), or right-middle lobe consolidation (aspiration).
- A referral for indirect laryngoscopy is needed for those with oropharyngeal dysphagia.
- A barium swallow may indicate an extrinsic compression, oesophageal web or diverticulum (all of which may be missed on endoscopy). Barium swallow also allows the assessment of a known stricture (e.g. carcinoma, achalasia, peptic stricture, radiation stricture) diagnosed with an endoscopy.
- An endoscopy allows direct visualisation of the oesophagus and biopsies to be taken, and endoscopic dilatation can be performed at the same time if necessary.
- A cinebarium swallow, using a medium such as bread or marshmallow, or oesophageal manometry may be helpful if the endoscopy and barium swallow are normal.

Further reading

Castell DO, Donner MW. Evaluation of dysphagia. A careful history is crucial. *Dysphagia*, 1987; **2(2):** 65–71.

Yang RD, Valenzuela JE. Dysphagia: a practical approach to diagnosis. *Postgraduate Medicine*, 1992; **92(7):** 129–46.

Related topics of interest

GALLSTONE DISEASE

Gallstones

Ten to fifteen percent of the general population have gallstones. Of these, 70–80% are asymptomatic, and only 15% will develop symptoms over 20 years of follow-up. 'Silent' gallstones require no intervention; those that do produce symptoms should usually be treated by elective cholecystectomy.

Several types of gallstones are described:

Cholesterol gallstones These account for 70% of all gallstones found in Western patients. Risk factors include:

- Middle-aged, overweight females, who have had children.
- Hypertriglyceridaemia.
- Oestrogen supplements, clofibrate or somatostatin analogues.
- High-fat, low-fibre diets.
- Certain racial groups (e.g. Pima Indians and Chilean Indians).
- Cirrhosis.
- 'Crash' dieting.

Pigment stones These are small (2–5 mm in diameter), multiple and tend to occur in an older age group. There is no sex difference.

'Black' pigment stones account for 25% of gallstones in the West and 70% of radio-opaque stones. They are probably caused by an excess of unconjugated bilirubin in the bile, which then forms an insoluble precipitate with calcium salts. Risk factors include:

- Chronic haemolytic diseases.
- Cirrhosis.
- Long-term TPN.
- Impaired ileal function (e.g. Crohn's disease or postsurgical resection).

'Brown' pigment stones occur most frequently in the East. They are soft, easily crushed and typically occur secondary to biliary infection.

Biliary colic

Biliary colic arises when a gallstone becomes impacted in the cystic duct or common bile duct and the gall bladder attempts to expel the stone. Attacks of severe (often non-colicky) epigastric pain lasting from 15 min to several hours are typical. The pain may radiate to the right-upper quadrant, back or tip of the right scapula, and is associated with nausea and vomiting.

Pain lasting for longer than 6 hours suggests the development of complications, e.g. cholecystitis or pancreatitis. Attacks of pain are interspersed by symptom-free periods of weeks or months (as compared with functional biliary disorders, where pain is felt on most days). Fatty food intolerance, postprandial bloating, flatulence and nausea are as likely to be due to functional disease as to gallstones.

Examination may reveal tenderness in the right-upper quadrant, but no peritonism. Blood tests may show the transient elevation of serum conjugated bilirubin, ALP and transaminases, but these do not necessarily reflect the presence of common bile duct stones.

Acute cholecystitis

Impaction of a stone in the cystic duct accounts for 95% of cases, the remaining cases being due to acute acalculous cholecystitis.

Acalculous cholecystitis occurs most commonly in the setting of severe trauma, sepsis or, more rarely, due to a gall bladder carcinoma, systemic *Salmonella* infection or systemic vasculitis. Such patients have a higher mortality and a greater incidence of complications, partly owing to the severity of the underlying disease.

Clinical features

Persistent pain (longer than 24 hours) in the epigastrium and right-upper quadrant associated with fever and nausea is usual. Murphy's sign (mid-inspiratory arrest due to tenderness on palpating the right hypochondrium) is typically present. Hyperaesthesia over the right hypochondrium (Boas' sign) may be present.

It is important to remember that in the elderly, confusion may be the only sign, and pain, fever and leucocytosis may be absent.

Mildly deranged liver function tests are present in 20% of cases – compression of the main bile duct by a distended gall bladder is often a contributory factor.

Imaging studies

All the following tests should be interpreted in conjunction with the clinical findings. No single test is diagnostic.

- An abdominal radiograph will reveal calcified calculi in 15% (but this is not diagnostic of acute cholecystitis) and, rarely, gas in the gall bladder lumen and wall (indicating emphysematous cholecystitis due to invasion by gas-forming organisms, e.g. *Clostridium perfringens*).
- Ultrasonography may show a poorly contracted gall bladder with a thickened wall, intraluminal echoes (suggesting stones, debris or empyema) and surrounding fluid accumulation. A positive Murphy's sign with the ultrasound probe is a further useful sign.
- The [99]technecium-hydroxy-iminodiacetic acid (HIDA) scan is highly sensitive and specific in acute cholecystitis. Radiolabelled HIDA is given i.v. and is rapidly taken up by the liver and excreted into the bile. The test is positive if

the gall bladder is not visualized within 1 hour, indicative of a blockage of the cystic duct.

Treatment

Most patients respond well with analgesia (e.g. pethidine, 50–100 mg i.m.), nil-by-mouth, i.v. fluids and i.v. antibiotics (e.g. ceftazidime, ampicillin and metronidazole), and are discharged for elective cholecystectomy.

Indications for immediate surgical intervention include:

- Generalized peritonitis.
- Possibility of other causes of an acute abdomen (e.g. peptic ulcer perforation).
- Evidence of complications (e.g. empyema or abscess formation).
- Emphysematous cholecystitis.

In the elderly, and in those with a high operative risk, the gall bladder may be decompressed and drained by the radiological placement of a percutaneous catheter.

Complications

Complications develop in 10–15% of cases. These include:

- Empyema of the gall bladder (mortality up to 25%). Cholecystostomy is usually the initial treatment of choice.
- Emphysematous cholecystitis. This is more common in the immunocompromised (e.g. those taking corticosteroids) and in diabetics, and carries a high mortality.
- Mucocoele. The cystic duct remains occluded by a stone or fibrosis, mucus accumulates and bile is resorbed, forming a chronically distended gall bladder. Superadded infection may result in abscess formation.
- Gangrene of the gall bladder wall.
- Perforation and biliary peritonitis (0.5% of cases, with a mortality of 50%).
- Cholangitis due to coexistent common bile duct stones (10% of cases).

Chronic cholecystitis

Patients present with recurrent attacks of biliary colic. Chronic cholecystitis is either due to the presence of gallstones, supersaturated bile and/or bacterial infection.

Investigations

- A plain abdominal radiograph will show 10–15% of gallstones.
- A fasting biliary ultrasound scan is accurate at detecting gall bladder stones >2 mm in diameter in virtually all cases. The cardinal features of a gall bladder stone are a mobile, echogenic focus with an acoustic shadow. In addition, in chronic cholecystitis, the gall bladder is thick walled and contracts poorly after a fatty meal.

	• In a small minority of cases, an oral cholecystogram (see below) or a ^{99}technecium-HIDA scan may be required.
Treatment	• Severe attacks are treated as for acute cholecystitis. Most episodes do not require hospitalization, and settle with a fat-free diet and simple analgesics.
	• Cholecystectomy is the treatment of choice in most patients with symptomatic gallstones. It has an operative mortality of 0.1% in those <50 years old and 1% in those >50. Complications include retained stones (in 2%) and the postcholecystectomy syndrome (approximately 10%, see below).
	• Alternatives to 'conventional' cholecystectomy are mini-laparotomy (through a 5–10 cm incision) and laparoscopic cholecystectomy. The advantages of the laparoscopic approach over standard cholecystectomy are a reduced hospital stay (1–3 days versus 4–12 days), a reduction in the time to return to work (1–2 weeks versus 6–12 weeks) and the avoidance of a long abdominal incision and associated complications.
The postcholecystectomy syndrome	This is the return of symptoms after the operation. The possibilities are that: (i) the symptoms were never due to gallstone disease; (ii) operative complications have arisen; or (iii) an unrelated condition has subsequently developed.

1. Causes. These include:

(a) Biliary
• Retained bile duct stone.
• Bile duct stricture.
• Biliary or ampullary tumour.
• Sphincter of Oddi dysfunction.
• Biliary dyskinesia.

(b) Non-biliary
• Peptic ulcer disease.
• Chronic pancreatitis.
• Carcinoma of the head of pancreas.
• Oesophageal reflux or dysmotility.
• Other (renal tract disease, IBS).

2. Management
• Establish if symptoms are the same as those precholecystectomy.
• Initial investigations include serum liver enzymes (serum ALP and GGT levels are elevated in retained common duct stones), endoscopy and abdominal ultrasound (note it is normal for the common bile duct to be slightly dilated after cholecystectomy – usually <10 mm).
• If symptoms persist, an ERCP is warranted.

- A few centres can offer biliary manometry for a definitive diagnosis of sphincter of Oddi motility disorders. Outside of such specialist centres it is hard to justify an endoscopic sphincterotomy for suspected biliary motility disorders, due to the high complication rate.
- An explorative laparotomy should be avoided if at all possible.

3. Treatment. If no organic cause is found, treatment for IBS or non-ulcer dyspepsia should be tried according to the predominant symptom complex. Symptoms may often be due to a motility problem ('biliary dyskinesia'), which may respond to antispasmodics or calcium channel blockers such as nifedipine. Some patients may need referral to a pain clinic.

Non-surgical treatment for symptomatic gallstone disease

At present, the following therapies are only indicated for those symptomatic patients who decline, or are unfit for, a cholecystectomy.

1. Oral dissolution therapy. Ursodeoxycholic acid (UDCA) (a naturally occurring bile acid which diminishes intestinal absorption of cholesterol) is most commonly used. The dose is 10 mg/kg/day in two divided doses. Mild dose-dependent diarrhoea is the only common side-effect. Only 10–20% of patients are suitable. Treatment is successful in 30% (probably less in obese/poorly compliant patients) and takes up to 2 years in those with gallstones of 5–10 mm in diameter. Stones recur in 50% of cases.
Criteria include:

- A functioning gall bladder, as assessed by oral cholecystography or ultrasound after a fatty meal.
- Non-calcified cholesterol (radioluscent) stones <1.5 cm in diameter (ideally assessed by CT scan).

2. Direct contact dissolution. Percutaneous transhepatic catheterization of the gall bladder and infusion of methyl-tert-butyl-ether (MTBE) dissolves most non-calcified cholesterol gallstones. It is an option for those who are unsuitable for oral dissolution therapy, but is labour-intensive for medical staff and is rarely used.

3. Extracorporeal shock wave lithotripsy (ESWL). Although the procedure is relatively safe and effective (after 1 year 70–90% of stones are eliminated), few patients are suitable.
Inclusion criteria include:

- A functioning gall bladder.
- Less than four non-calcified stones >3 cm in diameter.
- An accessible gall bladder and a thin abdominal wall.

Exclusion criteria include:

- Pregnancy.
- Liver disease.
- Bleeding diathesis.
- Cardiac dysrrythmias.

The patient is sedated (as for an ERCP) and positioned in the prone position. Shock waves are directed by ultrasound guidance to the gallstone. Several treatment sessions are usually required. UDCA is started a few weeks before, and continued for 3 weeks after, the procedure.

Complications include biliary colic (in up to 50%), cutaneous petechiae, haematuria and acute pancreatitis (in 1% – due to fragments obstructing the lower common bile duct).

Choledocholithiasis

In Westernized patients, common bile duct stones are of the cholesterol or black-pigment variety, and most originate in the gall bladder; however, they can occasionally form *de novo* in the bile duct after cholecystectomy. Although some common bile duct stones are clinically silent, most cause the following clinical problems.

- Obstructive jaundice (see 'Jaundice' (p. 180)) This is usually associated with pain, and if left untreated will result in secondary biliary cirrhosis and chronic liver disease.
- Acute cholangitis, characterized by pyrexia, jaundice and right-upper quadrant pain (Charcot's triad). Severe cases may be complicated by pyogenic liver abscesses and septicaemic shock. The only sign in the elderly may be the sudden development of confusion and lethargy. Recurrent attacks may lead to intrahepatic bile duct strictures and biliary cirrhosis.
- Acute pancreatitis.

Investigations

- Blood specimens should be obtained for full blood count, electrolytes, liver enzymes, clotting screen, blood cultures and group and save.
- An ultrasound scan is accurate in detecting dilatation of the common bile duct (the normal diameter being 2 mm plus 1 mm for every decade over the age of 20). Intrahepatic ducts are also dilated in more advanced cases. Ultrasound is relatively insensitive (approximately 60% sensitivity) at detecting common duct stones. Air in the biliary tree or liver abscesses may be present.
- A CT scan may be helpful in difficult cases, but often has little to add to ultrasonography.
- Endoscopic retrograde cholangiography and, in some centres, magnetic resonance cholangiography are by far the most accurate non-operative methods for assessing the common bile duct.

Treatment

- Adequate resuscitation with i.v. fluids, i.v. antibiotics (usually cefuroxime and metronidazole) and correction of clotting abnormalities with fresh frozen plasma and vitamin K is mandatory before considering any interventional procedure.
- An ERCP with sphincterotomy and stone extraction is needed as soon as possible if common duct stones are suspected. Very large stones (>2 cm) may be removed by mechanical lithotripsy (occasionally ESWL is needed). Temporary drainage may be obtained with an endoscopically placed biliary stent. Such stents can also be left in long-term, and used as definitive treatment for high-risk elderly patients with endoscopically unextractable large common duct stones. Immediate complications of ERCP include bleeding from the sphincterotomy and duodenal perforation. Acute pancreatitis develops in the first 24 hours in 2% of cases, but is usually mild and self-limiting.
- PTC allows visualization of the intra- and extrahepatic biliary tree, and, if necessary, the placement of a percutaneous drain as a temporizing measure if an ERCP is unavailable or unsuccessful. In patients in whom cannulation of the common bile duct by ERCP is not possible, a common bile duct stent can be placed. ERCP can be repeated using a percutaneously placed stent/guidewire to facilitate access for endoscopic procedures such as mechanical lithotripsy. In some cases stones can be pushed out into the duodenum via the percutaneous approach.
- Most patients with common duct stones require an early elective cholecystectomy. In those unfit for surgery (particularly the elderly), an endoscopic sphincterotomy with or without stenting may be all that is required.

Further reading

Tait N, Little JM. The treatment of gallstones. *British Medical Journal*, 1995; **311**: 99–105.

Related topics of interest

GASTRIC ULCERS

The incidence of benign gastric ulcers increases with age and they are more common than DU in the elderly. The prevalence of gastric ulcers is low before the age of 40. Females are affected more often than males, particularly if the ulcer is NSAID-associated.

Aetiology and epidemiology

Most gastric ulcers occur on the lesser curve around the incisura. The mucosa in this region is thought to be susceptible to ulceration due to its relatively poor blood supply.

Atrophic gastritis is a common coincidental finding, and may explain why acid and pepsin secretion in patients with gastric ulcers tends to be lower than in those with DU.

Predisposing conditions

- Although *H. pylori* causes antral gastritis, only 70% of those with gastric ulcers have *H. pylori* infection (compared with 95% of those with duodenal ulceration).
- NSAIDs cause ulceration by, amongst other mechanisms, inhibiting mucosal cyclo-oxygenase and thus prostaglandin E_2 production, the latter being involved with mucosal protection (e.g. by maintenance of mucosal blood flow and by bicarbonate secretion). Long-term use of NSAIDs causes ulceration (predominantly gastric) in 5–30% of patients and erosions and petechiae in 50%.
- Duodeno-gastric reflux of bile salts damages the gastric epithelium directly and alters the protective mucus-bicarbonate layer. This may induce ulceration in patients with other risk factors, but is unlikely to be a primary event.

Other factors

- Physiological stress can cause Cushing's or Curling's ulcers.
- Cigarette smoking increases the risk of DU, but has less influence on gastric ulceration. Smoking increases ulcer complications and impairs ulcer healing.
- Although various spicy foods are known to cause dyspepsia, none are specifically linked to gastric ulceration.
- Alcohol in high concentrations can cause gastritis and gastric erosions, but it is not a recognized risk factor for true gastric ulceration.
- The risk of gastric ulceration with corticosteroids has probably been exaggerated, and seems only to occur at doses of prednisolone above 20 mg/day, and in those patients also taking NSAIDs.

Clinical features

Gastric ulcers seldom present with 'classical' symptoms, and the severity of the symptoms are no indication of the severity of the disease. It is also not possible to differentiate gastric from duodenal ulceration on the basis of symptoms alone.

Symptoms may be absent and complications often develop in the absence of any preceding symptoms (particularly in the elderly and in those on NSAIDs or steroids).

- Epigastric pain is the most common symptom and it is frequently more severe than DU pain. Pain is not related to meals and may occur mainly at night.
- Dyspepsia is often episodic, following a cycle of 8 weeks of symptoms followed by 8 weeks of being symptom-free.
- Other frequent symptoms include abdominal distension and bloating, nausea and anorexia.
- One-third of patients present with complications, i.e. bleeding (in 25% of cases), perforation (10%) or pyloric outlet obstruction (typically leading to vomiting of food a few hours after eating). As for DU disease, the incidence of complications has diminished over recent years.

Physical signs are usually absent, but epigastric tenderness and a succussion splash (due to a gastric outlet obstruction) may be elicited.

Investigations

An iron deficiency anaemia may be found if the ulcer has bled (as with a duodenal ulcer). Features at oesophagogastroduodenoscopy (OGD) which may help to distinguish benign from malignant gastric ulcers are listed in *Table 1*.

Multiple biopsies of the rim and crater (at least six) are mandatory. Brush cytology increases the diagnostic accuracy to nearly 100%.

Management

1. General measures
- Stopping smoking has been shown to improve healing and lessen the risk of complications.
- NSAIDs and aspirin (even in low doses) should be discontinued if possible.
- Avoiding foods that exacerbate symptoms is appropriate, but specific dietary manipulation is not necessary.

Table 1. Distinguishing features of gastric ulcers seen at OGD

Benign gastric ulcer	Malignant gastric ulcer
Regular, smooth margin	Irregular, raised, nodular margin
Flat, smooth base often filled with whitish exudate	Ulcerated mass protruding into lumen
Normal folds radiate towards ulcer crater	Thickened, distorted folds do not reach ulcer edge
Usually <2 cm	Usually >2 cm
Heal with medical treatment	Rarely heal with medical treatment
May occur with a duodenal ulcer	Concomitant duodenal ulcer very rare

2. *Medical management*
- *H. pylori* eradication therapy should be given to those with proven infection.
- H_2 receptor antagonists (e.g. cimetidine (800 mg daily) or ranitidine (300 mg daily)) are effective. Ranitidine has largely superseded cimetidine as it has fewer adverse effects (<5% have minor adverse effects) and drug interactions. Ranitidine, at a dose of 300 mg at night or 150 mg twice daily, has been shown to produce a healing rate of 90%. Continuing treatment for 12 weeks has been shown to heal almost all ulcers.
- The proton pump inhibitor omeprazole has a superior healing rate compared to the H_2 receptor antagonists. At a dose of 40 mg/day before the morning meal, a healing rate of up to 96% has been found at 8 weeks.
- Uncomplicated NSAID-induced ulcers should be treated with a twice-daily proton pump inhibitor.
- All patients should undergo a repeat endoscopy after 8 weeks of treatment. If *H. pylori* eradication treatment has been given, repeat rapid urease biopsies should be taken from the antrum and body.

  If the ulcer has healed, biopsies from the site should be taken, as some malignant ulcers can undergo complete macroscopic resolution with acid-suppression therapy. If the ulcer is still present, the dose of H_2 receptor antagonist should be doubled or a proton pump inhibitor started.

  An endoscopy should be repeated after a further 4–8 weeks. If the ulcer persists after this second course of treatment, a carcinoma should be suspected, and a surgical procedure considered.

3. *Maintenance treatment*
- Without maintenance therapy, almost two-thirds of gastric ulcers without a correctable cause recur in under 1 year.
- H_2 receptor antagonists have been most widely used and they appear safe for long-term use. Prolonged medically induced achlorhydria (particularly with proton pump inhibitors) is associated with bacterial colonization of the stomach and the potential risk of carcinogenesis (see 'Dyspepsia' (p. 92)). For this reason the lowest possible dose should be used for maintenance therapy (e.g. ranitidine 150 mg/day or lansoprazole 15 mg/day).
- Misoprostol reduces the risk of complications in those who have had a previous NSAID-induced ulcer.
- Sucralfate may be used as an alternative or add-in agent.
- Patients most likely to benefit from maintenance therapy include:

Those who relapse soon after initial healing.
Patients (particularly the elderly) with underlying medical illnesses which would render them a poor anaesthetic risk if surgery is needed.
Those who remain on long-term NSAIDs.
Those with large ulcers (>2 cm).

4. *Surgical treatment.* Indications include:
- Malignant or premalignant change in biopsy specimens.
- Complications (bleeding, perforation or gastric outlet obstruction from a prepyloric ulcer or pyloric stenosis).
- Failure to heal after at least 12 weeks of medical treatment.
- Frequent and early relapse.

The Billroth 1 partial gastrectomy is most commonly performed. It is associated with a 4% mortality rate (for elective and emergency operations) and an ulcer recurrence rate of 2%.

Atypical ulcers
- Giant ulcers are greater than 2 cm and occur more frequently in the elderly, those on NSAIDs and those in end-stage renal failure. They take longer to heal and are more likely to be malignant.
- Prepyloric ulcers have a high incidence of complications (e.g. pyloric stenosis) and an increased tendency to recur on maintenance therapy.

Further reading

Peura DA. Proceedings of a symposium. *Helicobacter pylori*: from theory to practice. *American Journal of Medicine*, 1996; **100(5A):** 1S–64S.
Soll AH. Consensus statement. Medical treatment of peptic ulcer disease. Practice guidelines. *Journal of the American Medical Association*, 1996; **275:** 622–9.

Related topics of interest

Duodenal ulcers (p. 86)
Dyspepsia (p. 92)
Helicobacter pylori (p. 145)

GASTRITIS AND DUODENITIS

Gastritis

Inflammation of the gastric mucosa (gastritis) is either acute or chronic. For purposes of classification, the stomach is divided into two regions: body and antrum. Gastritis may predominantly involve one of these regions, or both (pangastritis). The nature of gastritis (bacterial, autoimmmune, etc.) can only be reliably diagnosed histologically, with biopsies taken from both the body and the antrum to assess the extent. Neither the symptoms nor the macroscopic changes at endoscopy are a reliable indicator of the severity or extent of involvement.

Helicobacter pylori gastritis is mentioned here but is covered more fully in 'Helicobacter pylori' (p. 145).

Acute gastritis

The term 'acute gastritis' is usually reserved for acute erosive conditions that typically result in necrosis and haemorrhage of the mucosa with relatively little inflammation.

1. Causes
- Drugs. Aspirin and other NSAIDs, cytotoxic agents or alcohol cause gastric mucosal damage in a dose-dependent manner.
- Infections. Staphylococcal and other bacteria cause acute bacterial gastroenteritis. Suppurative gastritis occurs in those with a pre-existing carcinoma or ulcer. It is caused by full-thickness invasion of the stomach wall by gut organisms (usually Gram-positive cocci or Gram-negative rods). *H. pylori* infection results in an antral gastritis, but this is seldom diagnosed in the acute phase.
- Caustic substances. Accidental or deliberate ingestion of noxious agents such as acids, alkalines (e.g. caustic soda, bleach) or industrial agents (e.g. formaldehyde) causes acute corrosive oesophagitis and gastritis. Important complications include oesophageal stricture, gastric perforation and pyloric stenosis.
- Radiation injury. Radiotherapy results in mucosal erythema and friability, superficial ulceration, telangiectasia, prominent rugal folds and antral narrowing. Severe damage may lead to scarring, obstruction or perforation.

2. Clinical features
- Abdominal pain, nausea, vomiting and haematemesis may occur soon after exposure.
- Symptoms usually settle within hours or days, and recovery is usually complete.
- Findings at endoscopy may be divided into three grades:
    Grade I (mild): mucosal hyperaemia and oedema.

Grade II (moderate): erosions and superficial ulceration.
Grade III (severe): extensive, deep ulceration.

3. *Management*
- In most cases, supportive management with fluid and electrolyte replacement is sufficient to allow spontaneous recovery.
- An H_2 receptor antagonist or proton pump inhibitor should be commenced when the patient is able to tolerate oral fluids.
- Following acid injury, the use of large quantities of water or milk within minutes of ingestion may limit the damage caused. A nasogastric tube can be placed for suction and the installation of antacids. An abdominal and chest radiograph is needed to detect perforation. Careful assessment and management of laryngeal involvement is imperative.

Chronic gastritis

Chronic gastritis is defined as any diffuse chronic inflammatory process involving the gastric mucosa. It is by far the most common category of gastritis and incorporates a heterogeneous group of disorders. It is a common finding worldwide, particularly in those of low socio-economic status. The incidence increases with age and it is estimated that approximately half of those >60 years of age have chronic gastritis. It is believed that most cases progress to atrophic gastritis over many years, the significance of which is uncertain.

1. *Classification.* The Sydney system of classification was introduced in 1990 to supersede the numerous pre-existing classifications of gastritis. The system has a histological and an endoscopic division, as shown in *Table 1*.

2. *Aetiology. H. pylori* infection accounts for about 80% of cases, while autoimmune disease accounts for approximately 5%. About 10–15% of cases are termed 'idiopathic'. Rare forms make up the remainder.

3. *Treatment.* General advice regarding avoiding alcohol, NSAIDs and smoking should be given. Antisecretory agents are usually beneficial. *H. pylori* eradication therapy should be considered in those with proven infection and symptoms that do not settle with conventional treatment.

Types of chronic gastritis

1. *Autoimmune gastritis associated with pernicious anaemia.* Circulating parietal cell autoantibodies and intrinsic factor autoantibodies occur in pernicious anaemia. These lead to chronic atrophic gastritis of the body of the stomach (sparing the antrum), achlorhydria, hypergastrinaemia and eventually malabsorption of vitamin B_{12}. Patients have a three- to four-fold increased risk of gastric cancer and a high incidence

Table 1. Sydney system of gastritis classification

Grading category	Variables
Histological division	
Aetiology (prefix)	Acute
	Chronic
	Special forms
Topography (core)	Gastritis of antrum
	Gastritis of body
	Pangastritis
Morphology (suffix)	Graded variables
	Inflammation
	Activity
	Atrophy
	Intestinal metaplasia
	Helicobacter pylori
	Non-graded variables
	Specific
	Non-specific
Endoscopic division	
Topography	Gastritis of antrum
	Gastritis of body
	Pangastritis
Descriptive terms	Oedema, erythema, friability, exudate, flat erosion, raised erosion, nodularity, rugal hyperplasia, rugal atrophy, visible vascular pattern, intramural bleeding spots
Categories	Erythmatous/exudative
	Flat erosion
	Raised erosion
	Atrophic
	Haemorrhagic
	Reflux
	Rugal hyperplastic
	Portal hypertensive
Severity grading	Mild
	Moderate
	Severe

of gastric adenomatous polyps. Prolonged disease results in G-cell hyperplasia which may lead to the development of neuroendocrine (carcinoid) tumours as a result of chronic neuroendocrine stimulation. An association with other autoimmune diseases (specifically autoimmune thyroiditis, adrenal insufficiency and type I diabetes mellitus) is well described.

(a) Clinical features
- Symptoms are typically absent until features of vitamin B_{12} deficiency develop (principally anaemia, with subacute combined degeneration of the spinal cord less commonly). Dysphagia due to an associated oesophageal web may occur.
- Examination may reveal pallor, a 'lemon-yellow' skin pigmentation, glossitis, vitiligo, splenomegaly and signs of impairment in the lateral and posterior spinal columns.

(b) Investigations
- A full blood count and film will reveal a megaloblastic anaemia, mild reticulocytosis, leucopenia, hypersegmented neutrophils and thrombocytopenia.
- Iron deficiency (due to hypochlorhydria-induced malabsorption, occult gastrointestinal bleeding and increased gastric epithelial cell turnover) may coexist.
- Parietal cell antibodies are almost always present, but intrinsic cell antibodies are more specific.
- Serum vitamin B_{12} is low.
- Schilling's test establishes the diagnosis of pernicious anaemia. After an initial loading dose of 1 mg of intramuscular (i.m.) vitamin B_{12}, cobalt-58 (^{58}Co)-labelled vitamin B_{12} is ingested. Less than 10% is excreted in a 48-hour urine collection due to the absence of intrinsic factor for absorption. An increased level of labelled vitamin B_{12} in the urine is found after the addition of intrinsic factor to the ingested ^{58}Co-labelled vitamin B_{12}.

(c) Treatment
- Treatment is with a loading dose of vitamin B_{12} followed by 2–3-monthly i.m. injections.
- Follow-up endoscopy for gastric cancer is controversial.

2. Granulomatous gastritis. Most cases are idiopathic and may mimic adenocarcinoma endoscopically. Specific causes are usually secondary to a systemic granulomatous disease (e.g. sarcoidosis, Crohn's disease (only 1% have gastric involvement), tuberculosis, histoplasmosis, leprosy or parasitic diseases (e.g. schistosomiasis)). The histological findings reflect the underlying disease.

3. Eosinophilic gastritis. This is characterized by the infiltration of eosinophils and inflammatory cells into the antral mucosa, sparing the proximal stomach. Symptoms of subacute pyloric obstruction may occur, due to stenosis or infiltration of the antrum with inflammatory cells. Anaemia and peripheral eosinophilia are common (but not invariable). Other causes of eosinophilia (e.g. allergic conditions, parasitic infestations, polyarteritis nodosa, Churg–Strauss disease, lymphoma, metastatic carcinoma) are usually easily distinguishable. The cause is unknown and the treatment is empirical, and may include corticosteroids, immunosuppressants and antisecretory agents.

4. Collagenous gastritis. This is a very rare condition in which a thin layer of collagen forms beneath the gastric epithelium. The presenting symptom is recurrent abdominal pain, and at endoscopy erythema and nodularity are found in the gastric body. The cause is unknown, and no specific treatment exists.

5. Duodeno-gastric reflux gastritis. This results from the reflux of alkaline duodenal contents (i.e. bile and pancreatic secretions) through the pylorus and into the stomach. It usually occurs following surgery (e.g. partial gastrectomy or vagotomy), but can occur as a primary event in those with a patulous pylorus. The histological features are characteristic – an inflammatory cell infiltration, oedema and foveolar cell hyperplasia. Treatment is empirical, often with sucralfate. The risk of gastric intestinal metaplasia and cancer development is increased (particularly in the postsurgical stomach), and surveillance endoscopies should be considered.

6. Hypertrophic gastritis (Menetrier's disease). This is discussed further in the topic 'Menetrier's disease' (p. 201).

7. Lymphocytic gastritis. The endoscopic appearance may be normal, or thickened folds (often with small nodules with central depressions) may be seen in the gastric body. Histologically, it is characterized by an infiltration of T lymphocytes (mostly CD8 suppressor cytotoxic cells) in the epithelium. It is sometimes associated with *H. pylori* infection, CD (about 50% of untreated patients have lymphocytic gastritis) and gastric lymphoma (although there is no evidence that lymphocytic gastritis progresses to lymphoma).

Duodenitis

Inflammation of the duodenum (duodenitis) is usually diagnosed by the macroscopic appearances at endoscopy. In reality, however, the endoscopic appearances can be misleading; an erythematous, apparently inflamed duodenum may show no inflammatory cells histologically. Duodenitis may occur alone or as part of the spectrum of duodenal ulcer disease.

Aetiology	The most common cause is *H. pylori* infection. Rarer causes include infections (e.g. giardiasis, cytomegalovirus, tuberculosis), Crohn's disease, sarcoidosis and ectopic pancreatic tissue.
Clinical features	Symptoms are usually very variable and may mimic peptic ulcer dyspepsia. Some patients complain of dysmotility symptoms (postprandial bloating, poorly localized abdominal discomfort), and many may be asymptomatic.
Investigations	• Endoscopy may reveal patchy or confluent erythema or, in more severe cases, multiple superficial erosions with surrounding oedema. The first part of the duodenum is most commonly involved.
	• Nodular changes may also be seen in those with chronic renal failure.
	• Biopsies are usually not routinely performed and show a wide variety of changes which do not always correlate with the appearance at endoscopy.
	• Gastric antral biopsies for *H. pylori* should be taken.
Treatment	Similar advice and treatment applies as for duodenal ulcer disease. *H. pylori* should be eradicated if present, and acid-suppression therapy given for 4–6 weeks. Those with dysmotility symptoms may benefit from a prokinetic agent (e.g. domperidone or cisapride).

Further reading

Bartelsman JFWM, Tytgat GNJ. Caustic upper intestinal damage. In: Tytgat GNJ, van Blankenstein M (eds). *Current Topics in Gastroenterology and Hepatology*. Stuttgart: Georg Thième Verlag, 1990; 76–80.

Related topics of interest

GASTROINTESTINAL INFECTIONS – BACTERIAL AND VIRAL

This topic covers gastrointestinal bacterial and viral infections which cause diarrhoea or dysentery (diarrhoea with blood and mucus) in adults. Infections in patients with HIV disease and traveller's diarrhoea are covered elsewhere.

Bacteria

Escherichia coli

E. coli that cause diarrhoea are classified into five major categories:

- Enterotoxigenic *E. coli*, which are enterotoxin producing; they are a common cause of diarrhoea in children in the tropics, and in travellers.
- Entero-invasive *E. coli* invade the colonic epithelium without toxin production (similar to *Shigella*).
- Enteropathogenic *E. coli* do not invade the epithelium or produce a toxin. They usually produce isolated outbreaks, in nurseries, of non-bloody diarrhoea with prominent mucus.
- Enterohaemorrhagic *E. coli* (including *E. coli* 0157) produce summer outbreaks following the ingestion of undercooked meat (often hamburgers) or milk. Infection presents as watery, then bloody, diarrhoea, and is associated with severe abdominal pain and only a mild fever. Important complications are a toxic megacolon, the haemolytic uraemic syndrome (HUS) (a triad of microangiopathic haemolytic anaemia, thrombocytopenia and renal failure) and thrombotic thrombocytopenic purpura (TTP). Both HUS and TTP are fatal in the majority of cases in the extremes of life. The diagnosis is made by the detection of the organism or free toxin in the stool, or by the detection of serum antitoxin antibodies.
- Enteroadherent *E. coli* and enteroaggregative *E. coli*. Some strains cause outbreaks of diarrhoea in the West, or traveller's diarrhoea.

Most cases are self-limiting, and severe infections respond well to co-trimoxazole or ciprofloxacin. Severe *E. coli* 0157 infection requires i.v. gentamicin.

Salmonella **spp.**

Salmonella spp. are found widely in wild and domestic animals, water sources and foodstuffs. Infection is usually acquired from infected animals or animal products, and accounts for about 15% of infectious diarrhoea in the UK. Four clinical manifestations are recognized.

1. Gastroenteritis. Nausea and vomiting are followed by abdominal cramps and diarrhoea (profuse and watery or bloody), lasting for up to 5 days. Diagnosis is made by stool culture.

Treatment is supportive and antibiotics should be avoided in uncomplicated cases as this potentiates the carrier state. Treatment with ciprofloxacin (or chloramphenicol) should be considered in high-risk cases (see section on general principles of treatment, below).

2. Bacteraemia. Although bacteraemia is usually transient and clinically insignificant, a potentially fatal Gram-negative septicaemia can result, particularly in high-risk patients. Metastatic infection, e.g. endocarditis, meningitis and osteomyelitis (especially in sickle cell disease), may occur.

3. Typhoid (or enteric) fever. This is caused by *S. typhi* or *S. paratyphi* infections, which differ from other strains as they are only found in humans, and cause a primary systemic, rather than intestinal, illness. Incubation is 7–14 days; the first week is characterized by a swinging fever, relative bradycardia, headache, abdominal pain, with little change in bowel habit. In the second week, the fever worsens and splenomegaly and an evanescent centripetal rash ('rose spots') appear. The third week is characterized by severe toxaemia and gastrointestinal involvement, with 'pea-soup' or bloody diarrhoea. Profuse intestinal bleeding, cholecystitis and intestinal perforation are possible complications.

Metastatic infection following recurrent waves of bacteraemia may involve the lungs, kidneys, brain, meninges, liver, bone or joints.

Blood cultures are usually positive during the acute illness. The organism can also be isolated from the stool, bone marrow and urine.

Chloramphenicol for 2 weeks is the treatment of choice, but resistance is increasing. Alternatives include ampicillin (but it is less effective at preventing the chronic carrier state) and ciprofloxacin. A short course of high-dose i.v. steroids is given to those with severe toxaemia. Three negative stool cultures are needed to exclude chronic carriage of the organism, which should be treated with fluoroquinolones and, if necessary, cholecystectomy.

4. Chronic asymptomatic carrier state. This is defined as persistence of the organism in the stool for over a year, and is commonest after typhoid fever. Women and those with gallstones are most at risk (the gall bladder is the main reservoir of chronic infection). Cholecystectomy eliminates the carrier state in 85% of cases.

Shigella spp.

Shigella spp. are found only in humans; they are common causes of dysentery worldwide.

The initial clinical features are watery diarrhoea, abdominal pain and a mild fever. Three to five days later, the organism invades the colonic epithelium, producing bloody diarrhoea, tenesmus and a worsening pyrexia. The median length of symptoms is about a week, and prolonged cases may be confused with ulcerative colitis.

Complications include toxic megacolon, HUS and septicaemia. Patients who are HLA-B27 positive are susceptible to a postinfectious arthritis. The organism is usually readily cultured from the stool.

Treatment is supportive, and antibiotics should be withheld except for the elderly, those with comorbid diseases, severe cases, or those with *S. dysenteriae* infection. Ampicillin is traditionally the treatment of choice, but resistance is becoming increasingly common, and fluoroquinolones are now favoured in some areas. Nalidixic acid is the treatment for *S. dysenteriae* infection.

Campylobacter spp.

C. jejuni is the most important species, and is a leading cause of bacterial gastroenteritis. Most infections are acquired following consumption of inadequately cooked foodstuffs, especially chicken. The incubation period is 1–3 days. Infection may be asymptomatic or result in watery diarrhoea or overt dysentery, often with pronounced abdominal pain. Systemic features are common and include fever, vomiting, headache and myalgias, all of which may precede the onset of diarrhoea. Diagnosis is by stool culture. Severe cases should be treated with erythromycin or ciprofloxacin.

Yersinia enterocolitica

Cases are most often reported in Scandinavia, Western Europe and the USA, where the organism has been isolated from water sources and domestic and farm animals. Outbreaks and epidemics occur following ingestion of contaminated foodstuffs from such animals.

Enterocolitis is the most common manifestation and usually affects children under the age of 5 years. Diarrhoea, abdominal cramps and fever characteristically last an average of 2 weeks – far longer than for other causes of gastroenteritis. Mesenteric adenitis (which can mimic acute appendicitis) and terminal ileitis (which can be confused with Crohn's disease) present in older children and adults. Bacteraemia is uncommon, but can lead to disseminated infection (e.g. to bone, endocardium, lungs, joints) in susceptible individuals. Joint complications occur in subjects who are HLA-B27 positive:

- Reactive polyarthritis (associated with erythema nodosum and erythema multiforme).

- Reiter's syndrome (comprising conjunctivitis, arthritis and orogenital ulceration).
- Sacroiliitis.

The diagnosis is established by a positive culture of stool, blood and, if possible, mesenteric lymph nodes and peritoneal fluid. A stool culture alone is usually not sufficient, and the laboratory should be informed if the diagnosis is suspected, as cultures for the organism are not routinely undertaken. Serological testing is useful if the presentation is delayed for more than 2 weeks.

Tetracyclines or fluoroquinolones are effective for severe or complicated infections in adults. Antibiotic treatment has no effect on the incidence or duration of reactive arthritis.

Vibrio cholerae

Cholera is a disease associated with poor sanitation and the organism is spread through water sources contaminated with infected faeces. Person-to-person spread is uncommon. Humans are the only known hosts and those with hypochlorhydria (which occurs with malnutrition) are especially susceptible.

An enterotoxin induces the severe secretory, non-bloody diarrhoea ('rice-water stools'); stool quantities can exceed 1 litre/hour. Dehydration is frequently severe, and death may occur several hours after the onset. The organism does not invade the epithelium and causes no mucosal damage. The diagnosis is usually based on the clinical findings, but it can be cultured from the stool.

The mainstay of treatment is early and aggressive fluid repletion. Tetracycline for 3 days shortens the duration of diarrhoea and diminishes environmental contamination.

Bacteria involved in food poisoning

These organisms cause an acute gastroenteritis by the action of highly heat-stable toxins (either preformed in contaminated food or liberated after sporulation in the small bowel (as with *C. perfringens*)). They rarely invade the intestinal mucosa, and hence do not usually cause bloody diarrhoea or systemic features. Although the bacteria listed above can cause food-borne diarrhoea, the term 'food poisoning' usually refers to infection with the following:

- *Staphylococcus aureus* is found in reheated cooked meat, cream-based products or milk and causes vomiting, diarrhoea and abdominal cramps 2–6 hours after ingestion, lasting for up to 24 hours.
- *Bacillus cereus* produces vomiting and later diarrhoea shortly after eating reheated rice, or any cooked foodstuff kept at room temperature. Some infections cause delayed symptoms of diarrhoea without vomiting, usually

following the ingestion of contaminated ice-cream, meat or vegetables.

- *Clostridium perfringens* causes predominantly diarrhoea and abdominal pain 8–24 hours following the ingestion of cooled stewed or 'spoiled' meat.
- *Vibrio parahaemolyticus* infection is associated with contaminated seafood or sea water. The incubation period is longer than for most other infections (12–24 hours), and intestinal invasion may occur producing systemic features.
- *Clostridium botulinum.* Canned or preserved food are the usual sources of infection. The incubation period is 18–36 hours and a progressive muscle paralysis may develop shortly after the gastroenteritis. Antitoxin is needed to counteract the neurotoxin and penicillin is used to treat any remaining bacteria.

Viruses

Viruses are the commonest cause of gastroenteritis worldwide. Four subclasses of virus-induced gastroenteritis are recognized:

Rotavirus
This is the commonest cause of severe gastroenteritis in infants and young children. Adults are affected through contact with an infected child, through water-borne outbreaks, or by travelling to endemic areas. In the West, infection usually occurs in the winter months and may be asymptomatic or cause self-limiting watery diarrhoea for 3–5 days. The virus is detectable in the stool by electron microscopy or the ELISA method, although these are usually only used for epidemiological purposes.

Enteric adenovirus
This causes endemic diarrhoea in children under the age of 2 years. The diarrhoea is often severe and prolonged, often with vomiting and fever.

Caliciviruses
This group includes the Norwalk virus and predominantly affects older children and adults. They cause outbreaks of watery diarrhoea, fever, vomiting, headache and myalgias in adults, which lasts for 24–48 hours. The diagnosis is made by electron microscopic examination of the stool, which is usually only used for research purposes.

Astroviruses
This is a less common cause of self-limiting watery diarrhoea and abdominal discomfort in infants.

Rehydration and correction of electrolyte disturbance is the principle objective. Apart from rotavirus, there are no vaccines available to prevent infection. Prevention of the spread of viral gastroenteritis involves advice on personal hygiene, avoiding undercooked shellfish, and adequate water and sewage treatment.

General principles of investigation and treatment of infectious gastroenteritis

- Uncomplicated acute gastroenteritis requires no investigations. Investigations are only warranted for high-risk patients, when more than one person is affected (particularly if this occurs in institutions), or if symptoms persist for >4 days (particularly if there is evidence of haemorrhagic colitis).
- At least three separate fresh stool specimens are required. Formed stools are unlikely to harbour pathogens (but may be used if chronic carriage is suspected, e.g. salmonellosis or amoebiasis). Stool concentration techniques are sometimes used.
- Inflammatory bowel disease and ischaemic colitis are the main differential diagnoses of acute gastroenteritis. No test is entirely discriminatory; however, a raised platelet count is more suggestive of inflammatory bowel disease, and a high faecal neutrophil count suggests an infectious cause. It is important to remember that an enteric infection may unmask latent inflammatory bowel disease.
- High-risk situations include:
  Extremes of life.
  The immunocompromised (e.g. HIV disease, chemotherapy, hypoglobulinaemia, malnutrition, lymphoproliferative disease).
  Gastric hypoacidity (as in the elderly or malnourished) or postgastrectomy.
  Patients with a haemolytic anaemia (including sickle cell disease) or hyposplenism.
  Joint prostheses (in the context of *Salmonella* infection).
- The mainstay of treatment is the correction of fluid and electrolyte imbalance with oral, or if necessary i.v., rehydration. Dehydration may be underestimated in the elderly, and the high rate of atherosclerosis in this group will further compromise the diminished organ perfusion. Rehydration should be carefully monitored in the elderly to avoid fluid overload.
- Antidiarrhoeals should be avoided if possible, and are contraindicated in children. They predispose to toxic megacolon in certain infections and may prolong the clearance of the organism.
- The indications for antimicrobials are discussed above. In general, these should only be given for severe, identified infections, as indiscriminate use promotes the emergence of resistant strains.

Further reading

Gracy M, Bouchier IAD (eds). Infectious diarrhoea. In: *Balliere's Clinical Gastroenterology*, Vol. 7(2). London: Balliere Tindall, 1993; 195–546

Related topic of interest

Gastrointestinal infections – parasitic (p. 124).

GASTROINTESTINAL INFECTIONS – PARASITIC

Protozoa

Giardia lamblia

This is the commonest gastrointestinal protozoal infection, found throughout the tropics and temperate regions. It is particularly prevalent in the developing world, where it is a common cause of morbidity and mortality in young children. It is transmitted by contaminated food or water, and may cause water-borne epidemics in the West. Person-to-person spread may occur in institutions. Giardiasis is now a recognized sexually transmitted disease, especially if there is oro-anal contact.

Infection may cause asymptomatic colonization; acute watery diarrhoea often associated with anorexia, bloating and weight loss, usually resolving completely within 6 weeks; or chronic diarrhoea, associated with steatorrhoea and weight loss. The latter is more likely to occur in those with an IgA deficiency.

Three separate stool specimens should be sent for the detection of cysts or trophozoites by concentration techniques. These may also be found on a duodenal fluid aspiration or jejunal biopsy. A duodenal biopsy may show subtotal villous atrophy, which in severe cases resembles CD. ELISA techniques for detection of *Giardia* antigen in the stool are available.

Tinidazole (2 g) or metronidazole (800 mg three times daily for 3 days) are the treatments of choice, and may be used as a therapeutic trial. Second-line treatments are mepacrine and albendazole as a single dose.

Entamoeba histolytica

E. histolytica is endemic in western and southern Africa, and Mexico; 12% of the world's population are infected. Transmission is by food and water contamination, and person-to-person spread. Humans are the major reservoir. Infection results in one of three syndromes:

- Asymptomatic carriage – 80–90% of all infections (5% prevalence in the West).
- Symptomatic amoebic dysentery (acute and chronic). Acute amoebic dysentery presents as bloody diarrhoea, abdominal discomfort and occasionally toxic megacolon (similar to acute ulcerative colitis). Peri-anal disease and paracolic abscesses may mimic Crohn's disease. Chronic intestinal amoebiasis causes episodic, often cyclical diar-

rhoea which progresses to become bloody. Anorexia, nausea and a low-grade fever often coexist. As patients often remain reasonably well, it may be mistaken for a functional bowel disorder. Complications include colonic strictures and the development of an amoeboma (an annular mass of granulation tissue usually found in the caecum or sigmoid colon).

- Amoebic liver abscess. This is the most common and clinically significant extra-intestinal manifestation of amoebiasis. A liver abscess may develop during the acute colitis, presenting with a swinging fever and right-upper quadrant/shoulder tip pain. In half of cases, there is no history of a previous colitic illness. Complications are often life-threatening and include spontaneous rupture into the pleural or pericardial space, or the hepatic vein, with spread to the brain or lungs.

Diagnosis is made by stool microscopy showing *E. histolytica* trophozoites containing phagocytosed erythrocytes (non-pathogenic strains are not erythrophagic). Faecal leucocytes are usually absent, which helps to distinguish it from bacterial dysentery. Multiple fresh stool specimens are usually needed to make the diagnosis, as the trophozoites rapidly disintegrate outside of the host. Sigmoidoscopy will reveal small scattered ulcers covered with a yellow exudate. Biopsies from the ulcer edge or the exudate may reveal trophozoites. Serological tests are positive in >80% of cases of amoebic liver abscesses and some cases of amoebic colitis, and negative in asymptomatic carriers.

A liver abscess is detectable by ultrasound examination. Percutaneous aspiration of the abscess is not necessary (and may cause a pyogenic abscess), but if performed will show the characteristic 'anchovy-paste' material containing trophozoites.

Treatment with metronidazole (400–800 mg three times daily for up to 10 days) is usually successful. Following this, diloxanide furoate should be given to those with chronic intestinal amoebiasis, and for those with chronic cyst carriage. Surgery is required for complications of an amoebic liver abscess, and for toxic megacolon or colonic stricturing.

Other protozoal infections

- *Cryptosporidium parvum* has its major impact on HIV-infected patients. It is found worldwide, predominantly in developing countries, where it is a common cause of diarrhoea in pre-school children, and in Western travellers. The diagnosis is by microscopic identification of oocysts in stool specimens (multiple specimens are usually needed), duodenal aspirate or jejunal biopsy by Ziehl–Neilssen staining.

- *Microsporidium* spp. and *Isospora belli* predominantly cause diarrhoea in immunocompromised patients (particularly those with HIV infection) and rarely cause disease in the immunocompetent.

Helminths

Although common worldwide, helminth infections rarely produce symptoms.

Strongyloides stercoralis

S. stercoralis is predominantly found in the tropics and subtropics. Infection is acquired through the penetration of the skin by filariform larvae, which enter the venous system and travel to the lungs, where they develop into adolescent worms. These worms migrate up the trachea, are swallowed and invade the proximal small intestinal mucosa, where they mature into adult worms. These in turn release embryonated eggs which hatch into larvae and are excreted in the faeces.

At least half of infections are asymptomatic. During intestinal colonization, symptoms include dyspepsia (which may mimic peptic ulcer disease), intermittent diarrhoea, anorexia and weight loss. A heavy infestation may result in steatorrhoea and malabsorption. The hyperinfection syndrome occurs in immunosuppressed or malnourished patients when the hatched larvae migrate through the bowel wall into the circulation (autoinfection). This causes chronic diarrhoea, bacterial peritonitis and Gram-negative septicaemia.

Penetration of the skin by filariform larvae produces local irritation and urticaria (cutaneous larva migrans). Migration of adolescent worms through the lungs produces a cough, wheeze and transient pulmonary shadowing on a chest radiograph (Loeffler's syndrome).

Serological tests for *S. stercoralis* are positive in 80–90% of cases. Larvae or adult worms may be demonstrated in stool specimens (multiple specimens are necessary), or in duodenal fluid aspirates.

Thiabendazole is the treatment of choice. Alternatives include albendazole or mebendazole.

Trichuris trichiura

T. trichiura (whipworm) is found worldwide, particularly associated with poor sanitation. Infection is acquired through ingestion of embryonated eggs which occur in the soil. Most infections are asymptomatic. Diarrhoea may vary from being mild and watery to being profuse and blood stained, often with mucus. Rectal prolapse, clubbing and iron deficiency anaemia occur in severe, prolonged infection.

Diagnosis may be made after the passage of a typical 0.5 cm worm per rectum. Sigmoidoscopy will reveal the adherent worms; biopsies are usually normal, but may reveal granulomas. Stool microscopy is less reliable but may reveal the typical barrel-shaped eggs or intact worms.

A short course of albendazole or mebendazole is curative.

Other nematodes

- Hookworm (comprising *Necator americanus* and *Ancylostoma duodenale*), although not a common cause of diarrhoea, is one of the most widespread parasitic infections, with a substantial morbidity in developing countries. Filariform larvae in the soil burrow through the skin, producing a local inflammatory reaction – 'ground itch'. These migrate to the lungs via the venous circulation, where they produce pulmonary symptoms (a cough or wheeze). They travel up the tracheobronchial tree, are swallowed, and mature into adult worms which attach to the small intestinal mucosa.

  The predominant clinical feature is an iron deficiency anaemia, and in severe cases, a protein-losing enteropathy.

  The diagnosis is made by the finding of ova or rhabditiform larvae in the stool or duodenal fluid.

  Mebendazole or albendazole are effective treatments, and in most cases iron supplements are also needed.

- *Trichinella spiralis* causes a systemic febrile illness and transient diarrhoea. The organism is transmitted following the ingestion of undercooked meat and disseminates widely in the body, predominantly to skeletal muscle, and rarely to the brain. The diagnosis is made by the finding of adult worms or ova in a skeletal muscle biopsy.

Schistosoma **spp.**

These cause bilharzia and five species are recognized. The commonest are:

- *S. mansoni* is found in Africa (commonest in Egypt), Central and South America, the Caribbean and the Middle East.
- *S. japonicum* is found in Japan and the Far East.
- *S. haematobium* is limited to Africa.

Infection is acquired by exposure to fresh water containing the infective form of the parasite (cercariae). The cercariae reside within the fresh water snail (the intermediate host), are released into the water and penetrate the host skin. These transform into schistosomules in the subcutaneous tissue and migrate to the liver, where they mature into adult worms. Male and female worms migrate as pairs to the mesenteric venules, where males produce fertilized eggs (the cause of the chronic inflammatory reaction). Some of these eggs penetrate the wall of the intestine and are excreted in the faeces. The number of eggs shed are in proportion to the severity of clinical intestinal disease. In fresh water, motile larvae (called miracidia) hatch from the eggs and invade the snail, thus completing the cycle.

Acute infection is manifest about 7 days after exposure by a fever, myalgia, urticaria, hepatosplenomegaly and an eosinophilia. *S. japonicum* has a more pronounced acute phase, 20–60 days after exposure, called Katayama fever. Diarrhoea with blood or mucus may occur as part of the acute illness or be delayed for months or years. Severe intestinal involvement is associated with small and large bowel ulceration, chronic blood and protein loss, and is complicated by strictures and obstruction. Chronic infection may result in granulomatous ova-containing masses within the bowel wall ('bilharziomas').

S. haematobium, apart from colorectal inflammation, also involves the bladder and may present with microscopic or macroscopic haematuria, bladder stones or transitional cell bladder carcinoma. *S. mansoni* and *S. japonicum* are common causes of presinusoidal portal hypertension. Such patients present with recurrent bleeding oesophageal varices with preserved hepatocellular function. A liver biopsy will show granulomatous hepatic fibrosis.

Diagnosis is made by the demonstration of ova in the faeces or a rectal biopsy specimen. *S. haematobium* ova are detectable in morning terminal urine specimens. A serum ELISA test which detects specific antibodies is able to detect present or past infection in >90% of cases.

Praziquantel is an effective treatment for all species of schistosomiasis. A single dose of 40 mg/kg is effective for *S. mansoni* and *S. haematobium* infections, and 25 mg/kg for 3 days is used for *S. japonicum* infection. Treatment reduces inflammation and fibrosis and improves portal hypertension.

Further reading

Gracey M, Bouchier IAD (eds). Infectious diarrhoea. *Bailliere's Clinical Gastroenterology*, **7(2)** June 1993; 195–546.
Yamada T (ed). Parasitic diseases: protozoa and helminths. In: *Textbook of Gastroenterology*, Vol. 2, 2nd edn. Philadelphia: J.B. Lippincott, 1995; 2343–79.

Related topic of interest

Gastrointestinal infections – bacterial and viral (p. 118).

GASTRO-OESOPHAGEAL REFLUX DISEASE

Gastro-oesophageal reflux disease (GORD) is caused by excessive exposure of the (usually distal) oesophagus to acid (and/or bile) refluxed from the stomach. In a classical case, the diagnosis may be made from the history or endoscopic findings. The most reliable diagnostic tool is 24-hour oesophageal pH monitoring, but this is too expensive to consider in most cases in such a common disease. Acid refluxing from the stomach may cause laryngeal and airways symptoms too.

There is some reflux of acid into the oesophagus each day in all subjects; in those without GORD this is mostly caused by periods of transient lower oesophageal sphincter relaxation (TLOR) not associated with swallowing. In patients with GORD, TLOR accounts for about two-thirds of the episodes of reflux, the rest being due to spontaneous or pressure-stress-induced reflux of contents across a lower oesophageal sphincter (LOS) with a lax resting tone.

Several factors increase the likelihood of developing GORD:

- Fatty meals cause delayed gastric emptying and transient relaxation of the LOS.
- A hiatus hernia may serve as a reservoir for gastric acid, increasing the likelihood of reflux when the sphincter transiently relaxes, and moves the high-pressure zone of the LOS away from the diaphragm, so that these two normal mechanisms for helping to prevent reflux cannot act together.
- Certain drugs may aggravate reflux disease by damaging the mucosa directly (e.g. NSAIDs, tetracycline, potassium chloride, bisphosphonates), delaying gastric emptying (e.g. anticholinergic agents) or reducing LOS pressure (e.g. theophylline, calcium channel blockers, progesterone).
- Obesity, tight-fitting garments, recumbency, large meals and an excessive alcohol intake may all predispose to GORD.
- Previous gastric surgery may cause duodeno-gastric and oesophageal reflux of alkaline bile and pancreatic fluid.

The extent of damage to the oesophageal mucosa depends on the duration of contact; the efficiency of oesophageal peristalsis and salivary neutralization; the composition of the refluxing acid, bile salts and pepsin; and the intrinsic resistance of the mucosa to damage.

Clinical features

- Patients complain of a burning and/or rising retrosternal discomfort (heartburn), often accompanied by reflux of gastric secretions into the mouth.
- Symptoms are typically relieved temporarily by antacids. Patients with functional reflux symptoms (see 'Dyspepsia' (p. 92)) usually do not respond to acid-suppression therapy, which helps to distinguish it from organic GORD.
- Pain may be associated with excess salivation.
- Acid reflux may cause oesophageal spasm, producing atypical pain which may simulate angina.
- Water brash, which means the regurgitation of acid or bile into the mouth.
- Patients occasionally complain of an unproductive cough, wheeze (nocturnal asthma), hoarseness or a continual need

to clear the throat, which may be due to reflux affecting the larynx.

- Odynophagia (painful swallowing) usually signifies oesophagitis or a stricture (when dysphagia is also present).
- GORD and oesophagitis may be asymptomatic, and the mechanisms whereby some patients experience symptoms and others do not remain poorly understood.

Diagnosis

- Organic GORD is reasonably reliably diagnosed on the history (there is approximately a 70% positive predictive value of classical features on history). A therapeutic trial of acid-suppression therapy for 2–4 weeks may helps to confirm the diagnosis.
- Patients with complicated heartburn (i.e. those with warning signs) should have an endoscopy before any therapeutic trial. Patients with dysphagia require an early barium swallow or endoscopy.
- It is important to stress that the appearances at endoscopy do not necessarily reflect the severity of GORD, and patients with severe symptoms may have a normal-looking oesophageal mucosa, and vice versa. Biopsies will usually show characteristic changes of reflux disease in organic GORD, but will be normal in functional disease.
- If the endoscopy shows macroscopic evidence of GORD and the patient is not immunocompromised, treatment may be started without the need for a biopsy. If Barrett's oesophagus (p. 22) is found, four-quadrant biopsies should be taken to exclude any dysplasia. If the patient is immunocompromised (e.g. HIV disease (p. 169)), a biopsy for histology and culture should be taken.

Ambulatory pH monitoring and oesophageal manometry

pH monitoring involves the transnasal placement of a pH probe 5 cm above the lower oesophageal sphincter (as determined by prior oesophageal manometry). The patient undertakes normal activities for 24 hours and the pH measurements are recorded (and correlated with symptoms) by a small device worn around the waist.

The British Society of Gastroenterology (BSG) guidelines for pH monitoring are:

- The definitive diagnosis of GORD in those with suggestive symptoms but a normal endoscopy.
- To confirm GORD as a cause for atypical symptoms (e.g. angina-type chest pain, respiratory or laryngeal symptoms), when the relevant investigations have been normal.
- When established GORD responds poorly to medical treatment, and particularly if surgery is contemplated.
- In the assessment of complex oesophageal disorders.

pH monitoring is *not* indicated as a first-line investigation in patients with atypical GORD symptoms, nor for patients in whom the diagnosis is reasonably certain and who have a reasonable response to treatment.

In the setting of GORD, oesophageal manometry is used to establish the position of the electrode for pH monitoring, and for assessment prior to surgery. It is *not* useful in the diagnosis of GORD.

Treatment modalities

1. Lifestyle modifications. Elevating the head of the bed by 6 inches produces subjective and objective improvement comparable to treatment with H_2 receptor antagonists. Other important lifestyle changes include weight reduction if overweight (a reduced intake of fat seems to be the most important factor), stopping smoking, avoiding late evening meals (particularly chocolate snacks), reducing alcohol and coffee intake, avoiding spicy or acidic foods and avoiding tight, constricting garments. Medication which may exacerbate GORD (see above) should be avoided.

2. Medical treatment
- Antacids and alginates. Antacids are effective in mild cases. They are safe and well tolerated with a swift onset of action which is short lived. Alginates (e.g. Gaviscon), taken after meals and at bedtime, form a viscous raft on top of the gastric contents, impeding reflux.
- Antisecretory agents. H_2 receptor antagonists (e.g. ranitidine 150 mg twice daily) relieve heartburn in 50% of patients at 4 weeks and heal moderate oesophagitis in 30% at 4 weeks. Proton pump inhibitors (e.g. omeprazole 20 mg daily or lansoprazole 30 mg daily) are more effective than H_2 receptor antagonists at relieving symptoms and healing all grades of oesophagitis.
- Prokinetic agents. Metoclopramide and domperidone increase LOS tone and increase oesophageal and gastric emptying. They improve symptoms of reflux about as effectively as H_2 receptor antagonists but do not heal oesophagitis. Cisapride produces similar effects by promoting the release of acetylcholine in the myenteric plexus. It is as effective as the H_2 receptor antagonists in relieving symptoms and promoting healing in mild oesophagitis. The main side-effects are diarrhoea and abdominal cramps, which are usually ameliorated with a gradual introduction. It may result in ventricular dysrythmias in those with a cardiac history and those on certain medications, particularly antifungal agents (check with the BNF or equivalent for interactions).

Suggested treatment regimen

- For mild intermittent reflux, lifestyle changes and antacids or H_2 receptor antagonists are usually sufficient.
- For more severe cases, a proton pump inhibitor should be supplemented in place of an H_2 receptor antagonist (e.g. a daily dose of omeprazole 20 mg or lansoprazole 30 mg or pantoprazole 40 mg).
- In more severe cases (persistent symptoms or moderate erosive oesophagitis), a higher strength proton pump inhibitor may be tried (e.g. omeprazole 40 mg daily) with or without a prokinetic agent.

After the initial treatment, patients should be maintained on the minimum therapy which relieves their symptoms. Unfortunately, the symptoms rarely resolve completely, and most patients require medication intermittently over long periods of time. Omeprazole (10–20 mg daily) or lansoprazole (15–30 mg daily) provide effective maintenance. Proton pump inhibitors cause hypergastrinaemia, reduce the ability of the stomach to sterilize its contents and, in patients with *H. pylori* gastritis, increase inflammation in the gastric body. There is, therefore, some concern over the long-term safety of these drugs, which should perhaps influence the management of younger patients with GORD with a lower threshold for surgical management.

For those with peptic oesophageal strictures, maintenance therapy with a proton pump inhibitor has been shown to improve symptoms and reduce the need for recurrent dilatations.

Surgical treatment of GORD

Surgical treatment should be considered for those with severe symptoms despite maximal medical treatment and for young patients requiring long-term treatment. The Nissen fundoplication is the procedure most often performed. Laparoscopic antireflux procedures show promise, but one recently published series reported a 1% mortality rate.

Reflux-induced pulmonary and oro-laryngeal disease

- Acid may reflux to the larynx, producing a dry cough, hoarseness or a continual discomfort, often with few other symptoms of reflux. Laryngoscopy may show white plaques on the posterior laryngeal wall and, in severe cases, ulceration and polyps on the vocal cords. Studies using pH probes at the level of the upper oesophageal sphincter may help to confirm the diagnosis, and treatment with omeprazole should be tried with laryngoscopy follow-up to assess the response to treatment.
- Evidence is accumulating that severe GORD may induce bronchoconstriction by vagally mediated pathways in the larynx. This is thought to be one of the mechanisms responsible for nocturnal asthma in children with GORD.

- Rarely, chronic GORD may result in direct aspiration into the lungs producing pulmonary fibrosis.
- Halitosis, dysguesia (a sensation of a bad taste in the mouth) and erosive dental disease may be further consequences of severe acid reflux.

Hiatus hernia

A hiatus hernia is present when the gastro-oesophageal junction is displaced into the thorax. It is a common incidental finding at endoscopy (often in obese women), and the incidence increases with age (30% of people over the age of 50 have a hiatus hernia). Two types are recognized: (1) sliding hiatus hernia – the proximal stomach moves up through the diaphragmatic hiatus (the commonest type); and (2) rolling hiatus hernia (para-oesophageal hernia) – the displaced portion of stomach moves through the diaphragmatic hiatus, adjacent to the oesophagus.

- GORD may complicate a hiatus hernia due to the fact that the relatively low intrathoracic pressure allows the reflux of stomach contents through the displaced gastro-oesophageal junction. Those with severe GORD usually have a hiatus hernia, but even large hernias may remain asymptomatic.
- Symptoms may also arise from mechanical obstruction in large herniae, strangulation of a rolling hernia (rarely), or from peptic strictures complicating GORD.
- The diagnosis may be missed with an endoscopy, and is most accurately made with a barium swallow (although this is rarely indicated).
- An incarcerated hiatus hernia appears on an erect chest radiograph as an air-fluid level behind the heart. The gastric air bubble may be absent. This is a not uncommon incidental finding in elderly patients.

Further reading

Anon. The medical management of gastro-oesophageal reflux. *Drug and Theraputics Bulletin*, 1996; **34(1):** 1–4.

British Society of Gastroenterology Guidelines in Gastroenterology (September 1996): Guidelines for oesophageal manometry and pH monitoring.

Epstein FH. The gastroesophageal junction. *New England Journal of Medicine*, 1997; **336:** 924–32.

Kuipers EJ, Lundell L, Klinkenberg-Knol EG *et al*. Atrophic gastritis and *Helicobacter pylori* infection in patients with reflux oesophagitis treated with omeprazole or fundoplication. *New England Journal of Medicine*, 1996; **334(16):** 1018–28.

Pope CE II. Acid-reflux disorders. *New England Journal of Medicine*, 1994; **331:** 656–60.

Spechler SJ and the Department of Veterans Affairs Gastro-oesophageal Reflux Disease Study Group. Comparison of medical and surgical therapy for complicated gastro-oesophageal reflux disease in veterans. *New England Journal of Medicine*, 1992; **326:** 786–92.

Related topics of interest

Barrett's oesophagus (p. 22)
Dyspepsia (p. 92)
Oesophageal dysmotility (p. 219)

HAEMATEMESIS AND MELAENA

- Haematemesis and/or melaena are indicative of bleeding from the upper gastrointestinal tract (UGT). The incidence is 80–150 per 100 000 per year. Bleeding from oesophageal varices, which accounts for 2–15% of UGT bleeding, is discussed elsewhere. An increasing proportion of upper gastrointestinal bleeds occur in the elderly secondary to NSAID-induced gastropathy.
- Acute UGT bleeding stops spontaneously in 80% of cases, but the overall mortality is 5–12% (20–40% in those patients who re-bleed).
- Surgical intervention will be required for 10–15% of patients.

Causes

The causes and approximate frequencies of lesions causing non-variceal UGT bleeding are listed in *Table 1*.

Table 1. Causes of non-variceal UGT bleeding

Cause	Frequency (%)
Duodenal ulcer	23
Gastric erosions	22
Gastric ulcer	20
Oesophagitis	10
Mallory–Weiss tear[a]	7
Erosive duodenitis	6
Carcinomas	2
Stomal ulcer	1
Oesophageal ulcer	1
No lesion found	5
Other[b]	3

[a] A Mallory–Weiss tear is a break in the mucosa within 2 cm of the gastro-oesophageal junction (usually the gastric side). It usually presents as fresh haematemesis in males, and often, but not invariably, follows vomiting and alcohol consumption.

[b] 'Other' causes are listed below.

Other causes of non-variceal UGT bleeding include:

- Watermelon stomach (or gastric antral vascular ectasia) which is characterized by spoke-like radiations of erythematous lines at the crests of the antral folds, radiating from the pylorus. The histological hallmarks are fibromuscular hyperplasia of the lamina propria and dilated superficial capillaries containing fibrin thrombi.
- Dieulafoy's lesion is an abnormally large submucosal vessel which protrudes through a small mucosal defect. It is characteristically within 6 cm of the gastro-oesophageal junction in the cardia or fundus and thus is frequently

overlooked. Patients (often elderly women) usually present with recurrent large fresh haematemesis.

- An aorto-duodenal fistula should always be suspected in a patient with previous aortic surgery or a known aortic aneurysm who presents with haematemesis.
- Haemobilia is blood loss from the ampulla of Vater and may arise following abdominal trauma, biliary tract instrumentation, or complicating a pancreatic pseudocyst.
- Angiodysplasia refers to a superficial dilated complex of arterioles, capillaries and venules. They are usually multiple, occur throughout the gastrointestinal tract, and may be associated with aortic stenosis and von Willebrand's disease.
- Telangectasia are areas of dilated groups of blood vessels which, unlike angiodysplasia, involve the whole bowel wall. They can occur in any part of the gastrointestinal tract, are usually hereditary and may form part of the Osler–Weber–Rendu syndrome.
- Other possible causes of upper gastrointestinal bleeding include portal hypertensive gastropathy and pseudoxanthoma elasticum.

Clinical assessment

A careful clinical assessment is needed to establish the nature and severity of the bleed. The aim is to identify patients at a high risk of re-bleeding and death, whilst simultaneously performing resuscitation procedures.

High-risk patients are defined by the following:

- Age >60.
- Comorbid disease (e.g. ischaemic heart disease, congestive cardiac failure, chronic obstructive airways disease, chronic renal disease).
- Those patients who bleed whilst in hospital for some other reason have a 20% mortality.
- Shock on admission is the single best predictor of severity. A pulse rate >120 or a *postural* systolic blood pressure drop of >20 mmHg indicates a 20% loss of intravascular volume. Frank shock (cold, clammy peripheries and a systolic blood pressure of <90 mmHg) indicates a volume loss approaching 40%. It is important to remember that elderly patients with ischaemic heart disease and those taking β-blockers may not exhibit a tachycardia.
- Bleeding from oesophageal varices.
- Continued bleeding necessitating >8 units of blood.
- Re-bleeding.
- Haemoglobin <8 g/dl on admission.
- Use of warfarin or NSAIDs.

These patients should ideally be managed in a high-dependency unit or ITU (although some studies have shown little benefit with this approach).

Other important features on the history pertaining to more serious bleeding include vomiting of fresh blood (rather than 'coffee-grounds') and the presence of haematochezia with haematemesis (which suggests an arterial bleed with the rapid transfer of blood through the gastrointestinal tract). Patients with a prior history of peptic ulcer disease have a 40–50% risk of re-bleeding. Elderly female patients with an NSAID-induced gastropathy are at increased risk of serious haemorrhage.

Investigation and management

- A size 14 or 16 gauge i.v. cannula should be inserted. A central venous cannula is not essential if good peripheral access is available. Such a cannula should, however, be considered for high-risk patients, and for those patients in whom the pulse and blood pressure are not reliable indicators of volume status (see above).
- All patients should have blood specimens sent for full blood count, electrolytes, calcium, glucose, clotting screen and cross-match (1 unit for every g/dl of haemoglobin below 12 g/dl). It should be noted, however, that in an acute haemorrhage the initial haemoglobin will not reflect the amount of blood loss, as 24–48 hours are required by the body to equilibrate the intravascular volume. The haemodynamic status is a better guide in such cases.
- Initial fluid resuscitation is with colloids, but it should be remembered that 1 litre of crystalloid or colloid prior to blood transfusion will decrease the haemoglobin by up to 10%. Blood should be transfused to maintain a haemoglobin of 10 g/dl.
- A chest radiograph, ECG and arterial blood gas analysis are needed for those with cardiorespiratory disease.
- Nasogastric tube insertion has been advocated in the past to detect the presence of fresh blood (indicative of active bleeding). This is no longer routinely performed due to the more rapid access to endoscopy, and the fact that such tubes may increase the risk of bleeding from gastric lesions and miss bleeding from duodenal lesions.
- In actively bleeding patients, the airway should be protected and aspiration prevented by suction, elevating the foot of the bed and, if necessary, endotracheal intubation and ventilation.
- Vitamin K and fresh frozen plasma are needed to correct a prolonged PT. Clotting studies should also always be requested if >4 units of blood have been transfused.
- Ongoing monitoring of pulse, blood pressure, urine output and central venous pressure (if necessary) should be performed hourly until stable.

Treatment

An endoscopy should be performed with 12–24 hours (within 4 hours if oesophageal varices are suspected). This will identify the source of bleeding, potentially treat the bleeding site, and provide prognostic indicators regarding the risk of ongoing or recurrent bleeding (see below).

1. Peptic ulcer disease. The endoscopic features and risk of re-bleeding from peptic ulcers are listed in *Table 2* below.

Table 2. Features and re-bleeding risk from peptic ulcers

Endoscopic stigmata	Risk of re-bleeding (%)
Active bleeding	90–100
Non-bleeding visible vessel	50
Oozing without a visible vessel	10
Red or black spot	5–10
Clean ulcer base	1–2

Of those who will re-bleed, 90% do so within 48–72 hours.

(a) Endoscopic therapies for bleeding peptic ulcers
Endoscopic therapy to stop bleeding from peptic ulcers is successful in about 80% of cases. Injection therapy, multipolar electrocoagulation, neodymium-yttrium aluminium-garnet (Nd:YAG) laser and heater probe are all equally effective, and the choice depends on the availability and the endoscopist's experience. A 'second-look' endoscopy is not needed when initial endoscopic therapy has been successful and there is no clinical evidence of further bleeding.

- Injection therapy. This is the most widely used modality in the UK, as it has the advantages of being safe, simple to perform, inexpensive and is readily available. The most commonly used injectant is 1:10 000 adrenaline. Other agents include polidocanol, ethanol, thrombin and fibrin glue (which consists of fibrinogen and thrombin). The method of action involves local tissue destruction, arterial thrombosis, vasoconstriction (in the case of adrenaline) and local tamponade. Fibrin glue is a relatively new treatment modality that causes the least tissue necrosis, and appears to be more successful than the other modalities if applied daily rather than as a single application.
- Unipolar or bipolar electrocoagulation. This modality involves the use of a probe containing electrodes which, when applied directly to the ulcer, generates heat and tissue desiccation. The main disadvantage of this method is that the probe has to be applied directly to the bleeding point, which is often technically difficult.

- Nd:YAG laser. Haemostasis is achieved by obliterative coagulation of bleeding vessels using a non-contact method. This method has the advantage of being safe and technically easier than the other methods, as no contact is required. The equipment is, however, cumbersome and not widely available.
- Heater probe. Heat is applied directly via a non-stick thermal cautery probe. This causes less tissue destruction than the other methods, and may also cause a tamponade effect due to local oedema. Some studies have suggested that this is better at achieving haemostasis in actively bleeding ulcers than injection therapy.
- Other therapies. Microwave cautery probes and arterial clip applications have been used in some centres, although their benefit remains unconfirmed.

(b) Medical treatment of bleeding peptic ulcers

Recent evidence suggests that high-dose omeprazole (e.g. 40 mg twice daily) decreases the rate of further bleeding and the need for surgery in patients with ulcers showing non-bleeding visible vessels and adherent clots (but not in those with arterial spurting or oozing). For those patients who are unable to tolerate oral medication, i.v. ranitidine is often given, but there is no evidence that it is effective at preventing re-bleeds. Somatostatin and tranexamic acid have been tried in the past, but have not been shown to be effective. Eradication therapy should be given to those with *H. pylori* infection.

(c) Surgery for bleeding peptic ulcers

The surgical team should be notified early for the following:

- High-risk patients (see above).
- Endoscopic stigmata suggesting a high risk of re-bleeding (see above).

The timing and nature of operation depends upon the cause of bleeding. Indications for urgent surgery are:

- Unsuccessful endoscopic therapy (i.e. continued bleeding).
- Patients who re-bleed after two courses of endoscopic therapy.

2. *Mallory–Weiss tear.* Most bleeds stop spontaneously and do not require acid-suppression therapy. Those that continue to bleed are treatable endoscopically in the same way as for bleeding peptic ulcers.

3. *Dieulafoy's lesion.* Injection therapy is usually successful, but needs to be repeated along the length of the submucosal vessel to completely obliterate it and prevent further

bleeding. A surgical wedge resection is an option for lesions which cannot be treated endoscopically.

4. Vascular lesions. Laser, multipolar electrocoagulation and heater probe have all been successfully used to treat antral vascular ectasia, angiodysplasia and telangectasia. Oestrogens (e.g. ethinyloestradiol) may diminish episodes of bleeding from angiodysplasia or telangectasia.

5. Gastric carcinoma. Bleeding is usually difficult to control and is often a terminal event. Injection with adrenaline and systemic tranexamic acid may be temporarily successful.

Further reading

Khuroo MS, Yattoo GN, Javid G *et al*. A comparison of omeprazole and placebo for bleeding peptic ulcer. *New England Journal of Medicine*, 1997; **336:** 1054–8.

Rockall TA, Rauws E, Wara P *et al*. Selection of patients for early discharge or out-patient care after acute upper gastrointestinal haemorrhage. *Lancet*, 1996; **347:** 1138–40.

Rutgeerts P, Logan RFA, Devlin HB *et al*. Randomised trial of single and repeated fibrin glue compared with injection of polidocanol in treatment of bleeding peptic ulcer. *Lancet*, 1997; **350:** 692–6.

Related topics of interest

HAEMOCHROMATOSIS

Genetic haemochromatosis is an autosomal recessive inborn error of metabolism, in which there is excessive inappropriate intestinal iron absorption over many years, causing tissue iron overload and damage. It is one of the commonest single-gene disorders. The genetic defect lies on the short arm of chromosome 6. Recent genetic studies have shown that up to 0.3% of caucasians are homozygous (and are therefore affected clinically) and 8–10% are heterozygous (these are carriers, having only a mild elevation of serum iron indices and not at risk of tissue injury). The mechanism of excessive iron absorption is unknown. Increased alcohol intake is known to increase the accumulation of iron in affected patients.

Clinical features

- Patients usually present between the ages of 40 and 60, and there is a mean delay of 5–8 years between presentation and diagnosis.
- Men are more commonly affected than women, as menstruation and pregnancy protect against excessive iron overload.
- Presenting symptoms are usually non-specific, and commonly include lethargy, diminished libido and hair loss.
- Examination may reveal slate-grey or bronze skin pigmentation, most marked in the axillae, genitalia and sun-exposed skin. Tender hepatomegaly is frequently found, but signs of hepatocellular failure are uncommon at presentation. The diagnosis should always be considered in a male with symptomless hepatomegaly and normal liver enzyme levels.
- The risk of development of hepatocellular carcinoma is increased 200-fold. This develops in 25% of those with established cirrhosis and may be the presenting feature.
- Diabetes occurs in two-thirds of patients and microvascular complications may be present on presentation. Diabetic control is frequently difficult to achieve.
- Anterior pituitary dysfunction affects two-thirds of patients. Adrenal dysfunction and hypothyroidism occur in a minority.
- Testicular atrophy is manifest by impotence, loss of libido, skin atrophy and loss of secondary sexual hair. In the longer term, hypogonadism may lead to osteoporosis.
- In 30% of cases, iron deposition in the myocardium causes a dilated cardiomyopathy, resulting in progressive right heart failure and dysrhythmias.
- Two-thirds of patients develop a specific calcium pyrophosphate arthropathy affecting the metacarpophalangeal joints (classically the first metacarpophalangeal joints) as well as the wrists, hips and knees. Radiologically, chondrocalcinosis is seen.

Investigations

- Liver enzymes are usually only deranged when cirrhosis is established.
- Serum iron is usually >220 µg/dl, serum transferrin is >80% saturated and serum ferritin is markedly elevated (but may be at the upper limit of normal in the early stages). Ferritin *can* be normal in the presence of hepatic iron overload, one reason being coexisting ascorbic acid deficiency. Conversely, alcohol and any disease causing an acute-phase protein response can cause an elevated ferritin in the absence of hepatic iron overload.
- Due to the inaccuracies of iron storage parameters, a liver biopsy is the standard for diagnosis. As well as the routine formalin-preserved specimen, some of the liver biopsy should be preserved in saline or equivalent and sent for quantification of hepatic iron (see below). Discuss the protocol with the local laboratory service.
- A Perl's stain is used to grade the degree of iron overload present in parenchymal cells in formalin-preserved tissue. The standard liver biopsy is also valuable in assessing the degree of cirrhosis present.
- A hepatic iron index (HII) (µmol iron/g dry weight biopsy divided by age in years) is highly accurate at distinguishing homozygous haemochromatosis from other causes of increased hepatic iron (e.g. alcoholic liver disease, chronic hepatitis C, chronic haemolysis, hepatic porphyria) which have lower hepatic iron indices. An HII value above two is considered diagnostic for haemochromatosis.
- CT scanning and, more accurately, MRI are able to detect a heavy iron overload but are not able to accurately quantify the degree of overload. They are sometimes used to assess the response to treatment with time. They can be useful in detecting hepatomas on the background of a diffusely abnormal liver.

Treatment

- Venesection of 500 ml is initially carried out twice weekly (500 ml of blood contains 250 mg of iron). The aim is a serum iron, ferritin and percentage saturation in the low-normal range. Once this is achieved, 2–3 monthly venesections of 500 ml prevents further iron accumulation. Patients should also receive folic acid supplementation and be advised to abstain from excessive alcohol.
- Diabetes may be resistent to treatment and is treated in the standard way.
- Gonadal dysfunction may require replacement testosterone and human chorionic gonadotrophin injections.
- Cardiac complications usually respond poorly to treatment.

- Hepatic transplantation is an option for end-stage disease, but is not as successful as for other conditions (principally due to cardiac complications and sepsis).

Follow-up management

Follow-up should involve monitoring of liver enzymes, iron studies and alpha-fetoprotein. A liver ultrasound should be performed every 6–12 months. A high index of suspicion should always be kept for the development of a hepatocellular carcinoma. These usually only occur in those with cirrhosis (about 85% of cases), and the risk is not reduced with venesection.

Prognosis

- Patients treated before cirrhosis or complications intervene have a normal life expectancy. Symptoms, precirrhotic liver histology and complications (apart from the arthropathy) generally improve with treatment.
- Untreated patients survive an average of 5 years from the time of diagnosis. Cardiac failure, hepatocellular failure, hepatocellular carcinoma and bleeding oesophageal varices are the usual terminal events.

Screening

The early diagnosis of haemochromatosis, before significant iron overload has occurred, is crucial, as early treatment will ensure a normal life expectancy. A candidate gene for genetic haemochromatosis has recently been identified close to the major histocompatibility complex locus HLA-A, and is termed HFE. Mutations of the gene are present in over 90% of patients with congenital haemochromatosis in the UK and Australia, but are only found in about 70% of patients with the disease in Italy and southern France. Environmental or other genetic factors may explain the disorder in those without mutation.

A simple test based on the polymerase chain reaction (PCR) method can now detect homozygosity for hereditary haemochromatosis. The test is valuable in screening family members, and in confirming the diagnosis in patients with raised iron stores. Those found to be homozygous should have a liver biopsy to confirm iron overload, and venesection should be commenced if iron overload is present. If iron overload is not detected, serum iron indices (serum transferrin saturation and ferritin concentration) should be checked every 6–12 months. A transferrin saturation of >50% with a serum ferritin concentration of >200 µg/l in men and 150 µg/l in women is usually is an indication to commence venesection. Such iron indices may also be used to screen all other first-degree relatives (beginning in their teenage years), and confirmation of iron overload then obtained with a liver biopsy. Heterozygous relatives should also be monitored yearly, and offered a liver biopsy if the transferrin saturation is >50%.

Further reading

Bacon BR. Diagnosis and management of haemochromatosis. *Gastroenterology*, 1997; **113:** 995–9.

Goldwurm S, Powell LW. Haemochromatosis after the discovery of HFE ('HLA-H'). *Gut*, 1997; **41:** 855–6.

Related topics of interest

Cirrhosis (p. 40)
Hepatic tumours (p. 150)

HELICOBACTER PYLORI

Helicobacter pylori is a curved micro-aerophilic Gram-negative rod with four to six flagellae at one end. The mode of transmission is unclear; however, it is often acquired in childhood, possibly via the faeco–oral route.

It is most common in the developing world and in lower socio-economic classes. The prevalence in the western world appears to be falling, possibly due to improved hygiene in childhood and a declining family size. As a rough estimate, the incidence of infection within the population in developed countries correlates with age, i.e. 60-year-olds have an incidence of approximately 60%.

The organism is of interest because:

- It leads to a chronic active (neutrophilic, and sometimes lymphocytic) gastritis in virtually all cases (spontaneous eradication is very rare).
- It is causal in over 90% of duodenal ulcer and 70% of gastric ulcer cases.
- It is associated with an increased risk of gastric carcinoma and mucosa-associated lymphoid tissue lymphomas (MALTomas).

Several adaptive mechanisms allow *H. pylori* to survive in the stomach:

- On initial colonization, it induces a profound, temporary achlorhydria.
- *H. pylori* characteristically produces urease, which catalyses the breakdown of urea into ammonia and carbon dioxide. Ammonia dissolves in water to form the alkali ammonium hydroxide, which neutralizes gastric acid.
- It possesses a proton pump which removes excess hydrogen ions from the organism.
- The flagellae provide motility into the mucus layer, away from luminal acid.

H. pylori and gastro-duodenal diseases

The relationship between *H. pylori* infection and clinical outcome (gastritis, ulcers, atrophy, etc.) depends on host factors (e.g. those with certain blood-group antigens, a positive family history and the male sex), environmental factors and certain bacterial factors.

Three different genetic loci have been identified for which strains harbouring particular alleles have a different propensity to cause disease. These loci are:

- *cagA* (the cytotoxin-associated gene which encodes the cagA protein of unknown function, but whose secretion is associated with more toxic strains).
- *vacA* (the gene which encodes for vacuolating cytotoxin).
- *iceA*.

In Western countries, a person colonized with a $cagA^+$:s1a *vacA*:*iceA* strain is more likely to develop a duodenal ulcer than a person harbouring a $cagA^-$:s2 *vacA*:*iceA*2 strain. These markers reflect degrees of risk and should not be seen as absolute markers of virulence.

1. Gastritis. H. pylori causes two forms of chronic gastritis:

- Most patients develop a mild, chronic active antral gastritis and remain asymptomatic. This is associated with increased gastric acid output and may lead to antral and duodenal ulceration (see below).
- Antral gastritis which spreads to involve the body of the stomach (where acid-producing parietal cells are found) produces a 'pangastritis'. This leads to atrophic gastritis, reduced acid secretion and hypergastrinaemia. This pattern of gastritis seems to predispose to gastric ulceration and possibly gastric adenocarcinoma.

2. Duodenal ulceration. H. pylori-associated antral gastritis is the major cause of DU – over 90% of those with DU are infected. A causal effect is suggested by the low recurrence rate of duodenal ulceration in those successfully treated for *H. pylori* and a high recurrence rate in those successfully treated with acid-suppression therapy but no *H. pylori* eradication therapy.

3. Mechanism of the pathogenesis of duodenal ulceration. The mechanism by which *H. pylori* gastritis leads to DU is not fully understood. Most *H. pylori* infections involve the gastric antrum, which contains G cells and D cells. G cells secrete gastrin, mainly in response to food in the gastric lumen. Gastrin stimulates the parietal cells in the gastric body to produce acid. D cells secrete somatostatin in response to acid, which in turn acts as a negative feedback loop by inhibiting gastrin, and therefore acid, secretion. *H. pylori* infection of the antrum in some way impairs somatostatin release from the D cells, which results in the unchecked release of gastrin and therefore increased acid output (especially in response to physiological stimuli such as food). With time, the increased acid load passing on into the duodenum induces a change there to gastric-type epithelium (duodenal gastric metaplasia). It is thought these patches of gastric metaplasia may be colonized by *H. pylori*, with the resulting inflamed, ectopic mucosa less able to defend itself against the high acid exposure, and duodenitis/ulceration resulting.

4. MALTomas. About 93% of MALTomas are associated with *H. pylori* infection. Normal gastric mucosa contains no lymphoid tissue, but infection with *H. pylori* results in a lymphocyte infiltration. A minority of such patients develop lymphoid follicles which may progress to MALTomas. In some cases, MALTomas have regressed with eradication of *H. pylori*.

Diagnosis of infection

1. Non-invasive tests

- Serological tests using the enzyme-linked immunosorbent assay (ELISA) method are cheap and simple to carry out. They are limited by poor specificity (50–80%) and have a sensitivity of 70–90% (depending on the commercial kit used). They are not useful to confirm eradication, as antibodies may persist for several months or years after successful eradication.

- The ^{13}C-urea breath test is more expensive than serology, but is more sensitive (97%) and specific (95%), and is mostly used to check for eradication after treatment. Urea labelled with ^{13}C is ingested, and the carbon isotope is released following the action of *H. pylori*-produced urease. This is detected by atomic absorption in exhaled carbon dioxide.

2. Invasive tests

- Direct urease tests (e.g. the 'CLO test') are performed during endoscopy, and produce a result within a few minutes. They have a sensitivity of about 95% at 24 hours and a specificity of 97%. The test is performed from an antral biopsy, which is embedded in a gel or placed in a liquid (depending on the particular kit) containing urea and a pH indicator. The production of urease by *H. pylori* converts the urea to ammonia, changing the colour of the pH marker. Acid-suppression therapy promotes proliferation of the organism in the body/fundus, and inhibits it in the antrum. In such circumstances, a specimen from the antrum may produce a false-negative result and therefore biopsies should also be taken from the body/fundus and placed in the urease test device.

- Biopsies may also be assessed histologically, and the organism identified on standard haematoxylin and eosin (H&E) or specialized (e.g. Giemsa) stained sections. This method is sensitive but expensive, and not specific (as other, similar-appearing bacteria are seen in hypochlorhydric stomachs).

- Gastric biopsies can be cultured in special media under anaerobic conditions; however, this also is expensive and requires technical expertise, and therefore is only usually used in research or to assess antibiotic sensitivities.

Treatment

Eradication of *H. pylori* results in healing of both duodenal and gastric ulcers, with negligible re-infection and ulcer recurrence.

Eradication therapy should be given to *all H. pylori*-positive patients with the following:

- Gastric or duodenal ulcers.
- MALTomas.

- Severe symptomatic histologically proven gastritis.
- Previously resected gastric carcinoma.

Eradication should be *considered* for the following *H. pylori*-positive patients (although the evidence for this is debatable):

- Non-ulcer dyspepsia.
- Non-steroidal anti-inflammatory therapy.
- Family history of gastric cancer.
- Long-term proton pump inhibitors for GORD.

Treatment of asymptomatic infection is probably not warranted on the balance of current knowledge.

1. Treatment regimens. Numerous eradication regimens have been described, and no one regimen is ideal. Any regimen that has a >90% eradication rate is acceptable; most consist of triple therapy comprising a proton pump inhibitor (which lowers the minimal inhibitory concentration of the antibiotics), a nitroimidazole antibiotic (often metronidazole) and a bactericidal antibiotic (e.g. amoxicillin, clarithromycin), taken twice daily for 1–2 weeks. The commonest causes of failure of eradication are poor compliance and nitroimidazole resistance. The latter is more common in certain population groups, particularly those who have received nitroimidazole antibiotics previously. In such cases, a triple therapy with amoxicillin and clarithromycin, or quadruple therapy with bismuth, should be tried.

2. Follow-up after eradication
- Those patients with duodenal ulcers who have had successful eradication therapy, as confirmed by a negative ^{13}C breath test 4 weeks after triple therapy, should not require long-term acid suppression. If symptoms recur and the ^{13}C breath test remains negative, a repeat endoscopy is warranted to exclude ulcers from other causes (see 'Duodenal ulcers' (p. 86)).
- For those patients with gastric ulcers, endoscopy should be repeated 6–8 weeks after completed triple therapy. This will enable ulcer healing to be assessed, cancer to be excluded (with repeat biopsies) and eradication to be confirmed (with a repeat urease test). For benign, *H. pylori*-associated gastric ulcers that have been successfully treated, long-term acid suppression is not needed. Recurrence of symptoms in such cases will require a further endoscopy to exclude other pathologies.

Future trends

Population studies have shown that it is likely that *H. pylori* is a 'normal' commensal of the gastric mucosa. With the declining prevalence of *H. pylori* colonization in the West, an increasing incidence of GORD and its sequelae (Barrett's oesophagus and adenocarcinoma of the distal oesophagus) has been noted. It is possible (although unproven) that these two observations are causally linked, and that in some way *H. pylori* infection confers protection against GORD. In the future, it is likely that we shall be able to test for, and selectively eradicate, only those strains associated with more virulent disease. Another likely development is of a vaccine against *H. pylori*, with successes in animal models already achieved.

Further reading

Blaser MJ. *Helicobacter pylori* and gastric diseases. *British Medical Journal*, 1998; **316:** 1507–10.

Tsai HH. *Helicobacter pylori* for the general physician. *Journal of the Royal College of Physicians of London*, 1997; **31:** 478–82.

Related topics of interest

Duodenal ulcers (p. 86)
Gastric ulcers (p. 108)
Malignant tumours of the stomach (p. 195)

HEPATIC TUMOURS

Hepatocellular carcinoma

Hepatocellular carcinoma (HCC) is the commonest malignant tumour worldwide, but the seventh most common tumour in western men. Chronic hepatitis B and C infection are strongly associated, and the increasing incidence of hepatitis C virus (HCV) infection in the West is likely to account for the increasing frequency of HCC. There is a large geographical variation in frequency, with parts of Africa and the Far East having the highest incidence. Cirrhosis (predominantly secondary to chronic hepatitis B virus (HBV), HCV, haemochromatosis and alcohol) is associated with 60% of cases of HCC in the West. It is hoped the increasing use of hepatitis B vaccination for susceptible people will reduce the incidence.

The frequency of HCC developing in a cirrhotic liver (from all causes) is highest in parts of Africa (>30%), whereas it is 10–20% in the USA and the UK. An increased intake of aflatoxin (a carcinogenic mould produced from *Aspergillus flavus* which contaminates nuts and grain) correlates with an increased frequency of HCC in various parts of Africa. HCC is a frequent cause of death in haemochromatosis, but is relatively rare in Wilson's disease and primary biliary cirrhosis.

Clinical features

The diagnosis may be made on routine screening of an otherwise asymptomatic patient with established cirrhosis. The diagnosis should be suspected in any patient with established cirrhosis who develops hepatic decompensation, right-upper quadrant pain or increased hepatomegaly.

Non-cirrhotic patients frequently experience right-upper quadrant or epigastric discomfort, weight loss, fever and non-specific constitutional symptoms. Jaundice is uncommon and has no bearing on the size of the tumour. Dyspnoea is a late manifestation and may be due to diaphragmatic involvement or lung metastasis.

Examination may reveal a liver mass, friction rub, arterial bruit (which is highly suggestive of an HCC but is also heard in acute alcoholic hepatitis) and ascites (which may be exacerbated by portal vein thrombosis). Right supraclavicular lymph nodes may be palpable, and signs of brain, bone and lung secondaries may be present.

Laboratory investigations
- Liver enzymes, particularly ALP, are usually elevated indicating underlying cirrhosis.
- Hepatitis B and C serology and serum iron studies should be checked. Serum ferritin levels are frequently raised in HCC, and do not necessarily mean iron overload or hepatic necrosis.
- Alpha-fetoprotein (AFP) is raised (>20 ng/ml) in 95%. The level correlates with the tumour size, although exceptions do occur, and a normal level does not exclude an HCC.

Serial levels are useful to assess the response to therapy. AFP is also raised in cirrhosis (the structure of AFP differs from that found in HCC, which can be useful in distinguishing HCC from cirrhosis); normal pregnancy; testicular, ovarian and pancreatic tumours; hydatidiform mole; and may be very high in hepatoblastomas. Levels are usually normal in other liver tumours, e.g. cholangiocarcinomas, fibrolamellar tumours and metastases.

- Carcinoembryonic antigen (CEA) levels are increased in liver metastasis, and may be useful in the differential diagnosis.

Imaging and diagnosis
- Ultrasound scanning is as accurate as CT scanning in detecting HCC, and is able to detect tumours <2 cm in size. Large nodules in cirrhotic livers may be misdiagnosed. Ultrasound is also useful for confirming the diagnosis with a guided biopsy, and for screening high-risk patients.
- Contrast-enhanced CT and MRI imaging techniques will give more accurate information on tumour invasion, the presence of satellite nodules and help to distinguish malignant from benign tumours.
- Hepatic angiography is useful to determine operability, and for therapeutic embolization and intra-arterial chemotherapy.
- A chest radiograph, CT brain scan and radio-isotope bone scan are needed if metastases are suspected.

Screening
Screening is indicated for patients at a high risk of developing HCC. These include men >40 years old with chronic liver disease (especially those with macronodular cirrhosis, chronic hepatitis B or C infection or haemochromatosis). Ideally, ultrasound liver scanning and AFP measurements should be performed every 6 months.

Treatment
- Up to 30% of tumours can be resected surgically. Criteria for operability depend on the specialist centre and the presence of comorbid disease in the patient (only those with Child's grade A or B (see p. 42) are considered suitable). Ideally, the tumour should be single, <5 cm in diameter, confined to one lobe and away from large vessels, and with no vascular invasion or metastases. The 1-year survival is 50–80%, and 5-year survival is 25–35%. Asymptomatic patients with Child's grade A liver disease, who are found to have an HCC on screening, have a 90% 1-year survival after resection.
- Liver transplantation is an option but the results are disappointing. This is partly due to the fact that advanced, unresectable tumours are usually treated and that postoperative immunosuppression enhances metastatic growth. Patients

who are hepatitis B surface antigen (HBsAg)-negative, with unresectable tumours <5 cm in diameter (ideally detected by screening or at the time of transplantation for another reason), have the most favourable prognosis.

- Hepatic artery embolization and/or chemotherapy infusion are used for inoperable tumours, but usually only with limited success. The hepatic artery is catheterized via the femoral and coeliac arteries, allowing the introduction of gel foam, and sometimes chemotherapeutic agents. Yttrium-90 microspheres have been used, which provide large doses of internal radiation therapy. The response depends on the size and extension of the tumour, the presence of arterial collaterals, the presence of a capsule and patency of the portal vein.

- Lipiodol, when infused into the hepatic artery (via the same route mentioned above), is preferentially taken up by tumour tissue. This is used in the detection of small tumours during screening, and as an embolizing agent as adjuvant therapy after surgical resection. Lipiodol-targeted lipophilic chemotherapeutic drugs (e.g. epirubicin) have been shown to prolong life in those with small tumours.

- Repeated ultrasound- or CT-guided percutaneous ethanol injections may be used to treat encapsulated tumours <5 cm in diameter. An improvement in 3-year survival has been reported in selected cases. The technique is also used to treat recurrent lesions and to control haemorrhage following tumour rupture.

- Systemic chemotherapy with mitozantrone may be used, but the response rate is poor.

- External beam radiotherapy is not effective.

Prognosis

Hepatic artery embolization, transplantation and surgical resection of early tumours all prolong survival, but the prognosis remains very poor. The median survival after diagnosis is about 3 months.

Fibrolamellar carcinoma

This tumour occurs between the ages of 5 and 35 years and is unrelated to cirrhosis. Most patients present with upper abdominal discomfort and a right-upper abdominal mass. Blood tests may reveal a raised calcium (due to pseudohyperparathyroidism) and the AFP level is normal. An ultrasound scan shows homogenous hyperechoic lesions, and a CT scan will show a well enhanced hypodense mass, often with calcification. Characteristic histological features are the presence of large, polygonal eosinophilic tumour cells with intracytoplasmic fibrinogen bodies, interspersed with bands of mature fibrous tissue. Distant metastasis is uncommon, although most spread to regional lymph nodes. The treatment is surgical excision or transplantation. The prognosis is better than for HCC – about 3–5 years.

Hepatic metastases

- In the West, 90% of malignant liver tumours are metastases.
- About one-third of all cancers metastasize to the liver, the commonest primaries being cancers of the stomach, colorectum, breast, lung, pancreas, oesophagus and malignant melanoma. Metastases are said not to occur in cirrhotic livers.
- The diagnosis is usually made by ultrasound, but contrast-enhanced/spiral CT and MRI scanning have improved sensitivity. Ultrasound- or CT-guided percutaneous biopsy is used to confirm the diagnosis, but is often of little help in determining the primary. Cytological examinations of aspirated fluid are occasionally helpful in this regard.
- Of patients with colorectal metastases, 5–10% are amenable to surgical excision (usually a lobectomy). Such patients should have fewer than four liver lesions, preferably involving a single lobe, an adequate resectable margin, no extrahepatic spread and no precluding medical conditions. Five-year survival figures of >25% have been achieved. Hepatic artery infusional chemotherapy significantly improves survival in those with colorectal metastases and may be used as an adjuvant to surgical resection.
- Metastases from breast cancer are sometimes treated with combined systemic chemotherapy with variable results. Arterial embolization with gel foam is used in certain circumstances. Radiotherapy is not effective.

Benign tumours of the liver

Haemangioma

- This is the commonest benign tumour of the liver and is found in 5% of autopsies. They are common incidental findings during ultrasound or CT screening. They are usually small, single (but may be multiple), subcapsular and located in the right lobe of the liver.
- Occasionally large haemangiomas produce pain (due to thrombosis), an abdominal mass or a venous hum.
- A plain radiograph may show calcification. Ultrasound commonly shows a small, solitary, well-defined echogenic lesion, with a characteristic posterior acoustic shadow. Contrast-enhanced CT and MRI scanning (the latter being more sensitive) show characteristic contrast enhancement. Hepatic angiography may be needed if the imaging studies are not typical. Inadvertent percutaneous needle biopsy of a haemangioma rarely causes complications.
- No treatment is necessary. Large haemangiomas that cause pain or rapidly expand can be safely resected.

Hepatic adenoma

These very rare tumours are associated with use of the oral contraceptive pill and with pregnancy. They usually present as a right-upper quadrant mass, or as an acute intra-abdominal haemorrhage, often in pregnancy.

Further reading

Saini S. Imaging of the hepatobiliary tract. *New England Journal of Medicine*, 1997; **336:** 1889–94.

Related topic of interest

Cirrhosis (p. 40)

HEPATITIS A

Hepatitis A virus (HAV) is a ribonucleic acid (RNA) virus spread via the faeco–oral route. Infection is usually self-limiting and may be sporadic or epidemic.

Transmission may arise in the following circumstances:

- Children, especially those living in overcrowded/unhygienic conditions.
- Sexually active homosexual men.
- Travellers to the Far East.
- Ingestion of contaminated seafood (especially molluscs).
- Contaminated food (e.g. fruit juices, salads, meat).

Clinical features

Incubation is from 2 days to 2 weeks. Most people are infected before the age of 14, when the infection is either subclinical or presents as a mild self-limiting gastroenteritis. In adults, an icteric illness is preceded by a prodromal illness of malaise, nausea and pyrexia. In icteric illness due to hepatitis A, transaminase levels are usually extremely high. Some patients may experience right-upper quadrant discomfort and tenderness. Onset of jaundice coincides with transient darkening of the urine, pallor of stools, and a gradual resolution of symptoms. Clinical examination will reveal jaundice, generalized lymphadenopathy, and tender hepatosplenomegaly, but no signs of chronic liver disease. Malaise and fatigue may persist for up to 6 weeks. Full clinical and biochemical recovery is usual within 3 months.

Occasionally in adults, the jaundice is predominantly cholestatic (pruritus being prominent) and may last for several months. Full recovery is the rule; prednisolone may reduce the duration. Hepatitis A (unlike B and C) may relapse 1–3 months after the original attack. The relapse is indistiguishable from the initial event, and full recovery eventually occurs.

Mortality due to fulminant hepatitis is very rare (<1:1000). Chronic infection does not occur.

Rare associations with the acute illness are the Guillain–Barre syndrome, the nephrotic syndrome and the triggering of chronic autoimmune hepatitis in susceptible patients.

Serological diagnosis

- Anti-HAV IgM rises 8 weeks after exposure and persists for 3–4 months. It signifies acute HAV infection.
- Anti-HAV IgG rises 1–2 weeks later and persists for several years. Its presence implies immunity to HAV infection.

Treatment

No specific treatment is necessary. Alcohol and potentially hepatotoxic drugs should be avoided. A low-fat diet is usually preferred by the patient, but this does not alter the course of the illness. All cases should be notified to the Medical Director for Environmental Health.

Prevention

HAV is shed in the faeces for up to 2 weeks before the onset of jaundice, and hence isolation of patients at the time of the onset of jaundice does not greatly affect the spread of infection.

- Passive immunization with i.m. immune serum globulin (ISG) is used within 6 days for those who have had close personal contact with a case.
- Active immunization with inactivated virus i.m. provides effective protection for a year. A booster 6–12 months later provides long-term protection.
- Those who would benefit from vaccination include:
  Travellers to areas of poor hygiene.
  Nursing staff in hospitals.
  Food handlers and sewage workers.
  Sexually active homosexual males.

Further reading

Sherlock S, Dooley J. Viral hepatitis. In: *Diseases of the Liver and Biliary System*, 10th edn. Oxford: Blackwell Science, 1997; 265–302.

Related topics of interest

Abnormal liver tests (p. 1)
Hepatitis B and D (p. 157)
Hepatitis C, E and G (p. 163)

HEPATITIS B AND D

Hepatitis B

- HBV is a deoxyribonucleic acid (DNA) virus that invades and replicates in hepatocytes.
- It sheds HBsAg, hepatitis B 'e' antigen (HBeAg) and intact virions (containing HBV DNA).
- The diagnosis of acute hepatitis B is made with a positive serum HBsAg and anti-hepatitis B core antibody (HBcAb) – both IgM and IgG. Chronic disease is characterized by the persistent presence of HBV DNA and HBeAg.
- Clinical remission is characterized by the disappearance of HBV DNA and HBeAg (the latter indicating a sustained remission), and the seroconversion to anti-hepatitis B 'e' antibody (HBeAb) positive.
- HBsAg may remain positive after remission but many patients eventually become HBsAg negative.
- Chronic hepatitis B accounts for 5–10% of cases of chronic liver disease and cirrhosis in developed countries.

Epidemiology

HBV is transmitted parenterally or by intimate, usually sexual, contact. The carriage rate of HBsAg varies from 0.1–0.2% in Western countries to 10–15% in Africa and the Far East, and as high as 85% in Australian Aborigines. In high endemic areas, transmission is both vertical (i.e. during birth) and horizontal (i.e. close personal contact in childhood).

High-risk groups are:

- Intravenous drug users.
- Male homosexuals.
- Patients requiring frequent blood transfusions.
- Health care workers – surgeons and dentists are particularly at risk.
- Patients of HBsAg-positive – and especially HBeAg-positive – surgeons who perform complex invasive procedures.
- Staff and patients in institutions for those with learning difficulties.
- Neonates of HBsAg-positive mothers.
- People from high endemic areas.
- Patients with renal failure on dialysis, lymphoma, cancer or organ transplantation.

Clinical course

Subclinical infection in adults is very common. Such non-icteric cases are more likely to become chronic than icteric cases. Acute illness in adults is usually more severe than that for acute hepatitis A or C. Incubation is 8–24 weeks. Five to twenty percent of cases are complicated by chronic infection.

A serum sickness-like prodromal illness occurs about a week before the onset of jaundice and lasts for up to 2 weeks.

Features include fever, malaise, nausea, an urticarial rash and asymmetrical small-joint arthropathy. Jaundice occurs when the prodrome starts to subside. Pale stool and dark urine are common, but prolonged or severe cholestatic jaundice is unusual. Symptoms usually last for less than 4 months and jaundice for less than 4 weeks. A severe course over 1–3 months with a high mortality due to subacute hepatic necrosis may occur.

Various extrahepatic conditions are associated with circulating immune complexes containing HBsAg in the setting of mild chronic liver disease. These include:

- Polyarteritis nodosa.
- Glomerulonephritis.
- Polymyalgia rheumatica.
- Myocarditis.
- Guillian–Barre syndrome.

Outcome

Anorexia and lethargy are common persistent symptoms after the acute illness, and a full recovery may take several months. Fulminant hepatic failure occurs in about 1% of symptomatic infections and is more common in the setting of superimposed hepatitis D virus (HDV), HAV or HCV infection.

Approximately 10% of adults (usually males) contracting HBV will not clear HBsAg from the serum within 6 months. The majority remain 'healthy' carriers, of whom about 5% per annum seroconvert to anti-hepatitis B antibody (HB Ab) positive, HBsAg negative. One to two percent of chronic carriers will develop serious liver disease including cirrhosis and hepatoma.

Serological diagnosis

- Serum HBsAg is present 6 weeks after infection and persists for 3 months. Persistence for longer than 6 months defines a chronic carrier.
- Most patients develop anti-hepatitis B surface antibody (HBsAb) about 3 months after the onset of infection. Its presence implies recovery, but not necessarily immunity.
- HBeAg is transiently present during an acute attack, but if it persists it suggests ongoing viral replication and continued infectivity.
- Anti-HBeAb rises after the acute attack and indicates a low infectivity and a strong possibility that complete recovery will ensue.
- Hepatitis B core antigen (HBcAg) cannot be detected serologically. IgM anti-HBcAb is present in high titres in acute infection and in low titres in chronic active hepatitis. IgG anti-HBcAb with absent HBsAg indicates past exposure to HBV infection, and with positive HBsAg indicates ongoing chronic infection.

- HBV DNA as detected by PCR is the best marker of on-going viral replication and hence infectivity.
- A small proportion of patients with chronic HBV infection are infected with a strain with a mutation in the precore region (precore mutant). Such strains do not secrete HBeAg, are associated with severe fulminant disease in some countries, and respond poorly to interferon therapy (see below). Numerous other mutant strains have been described, many of which may escape the host immune defences and cause fulminant disease.

Treatment

- All cases of viral hepatitis must be notified to the Medical Officer for Environmental Health.
- Alcohol and potentially hepatotoxic drugs should be avoided. A low-fat diet is often preferred by the patient but has no bearing on the outcome.
- Patients should be counselled regarding personal infectivity (especially those who are HBeAg positive). Close family/personal/sexual contacts should be checked for HBsAb and HBcAb and, if negative, they should be vaccinated (see below).
- In patients with chronic infection, interferon alpha (IFN-α) induces a long-term remission in a third of patients after 4–6 months of treatment. The current regimen for adults is 5 million units by subcutaneous injection thrice weekly for 4 months.

Optimum use of interferon in hepatitis B depends on an understanding of the natural history of chronic infection. Patients with chronic hepatitis B initially mount little or no immune response to the virus (the 'immunotolerant' phase). During this time, HBV DNA levels are high, but little damage is being done to hepatocytes – transaminases are normal/mildly elevated and a liver biopsy shows little or no inflammation. There is little point, or need, to treat with interferon in this stage.

After a variable interval of months to many years, immune tolerance is lost, and an immune attack on hepatitis B-infected hepatocytes commences. It is this host immune response that causes significant liver damage. A partially effective immune response does not clear the virus, but continues to damage hepatocytes, and may lead to cirrhosis, liver failure or hepatoma. Treatment should be aimed at minimizing the duration of this phase. The role of interferon is to boost the host's own immune response to ensure it is completely effective.

The response to treatment should be monitored with amino-transferase levels every 2–4 weeks and HBsAg, HBeAg and HBV DNA measured at the end of treatment and 6 months later. A beneficial response is defined as a negative HBeAg and HBV DNA, seroconversion to HBeAb positive, and normal or near-normal aminotransferases 6 months after the end of treatment.

Those patients likely to benefit from, and have a sustained respond to, IFN-α are those with (i) evidence indicating active host immune response to the virus:

- High serum aminotransferase levels.
- Biopsy showing active liver inflammation.
- Low HBV DNA levels.

and (ii) the following other features:

- A short duration of disease before treatment.
- Wild-type (HBeAg-positive) virus.
- Absence of coexisting diseases causing immunosuppression.

Adverse effects include:

- Flu-like symptoms 6–8 hours after injection; paracetamol is helpful to control this.
- Lethargy, nausea, abdominal pain, headache, myalgias, weight loss, hair loss.
- Neurological and psychological – confusion, seizures, vertigo, visual and hearing impairment, anxiety and depression (suicidal behaviour has been reported).
- Haematological – thrombocytopenia, neutropenia.
- Cardiovascular – hypotension, arrhythmias.
- Immunological – increased susceptibility to bacterial infections, autoantibody formation and autoimmune diseases.
- Thyroid abnormalities – thyroid function tests should be monitored in all patients.

As IFN-α is effective in only a minority of patients, other therapies are being sought. Famciclovir and lamivudine are new oral nucleoside analogues which are well tolerated. They are able to provide sustained inhibition of viral replication when used for prolonged periods in combination, or with interferon.

Immunization

Passive immunization with hyperimmune hepatitis B immunoglobulin (HBIG) should be given in the following cases:

- Sexual, or close, contact with someone with acute infection or high infectivity.
- Parenteral exposure (e.g. needlestick injury) to HBsAg-positive blood.

- Babies born to HBsAg-positive mothers.
- Post-liver transplant in a patient who is HBV DNA positive.

HBIG should always be given with HBV vaccine to prevent re-infection.

Active immunization with hepatitis B vaccine (which contains inactive HBsAg) should be used in the following high-risk groups:

- Intravenous drug users.
- Those with multiple sexual partners.
- Homosexually active men.
- Close family contacts of a case or carrier.
- Infants born to affected mothers.
- All health care workers (including doctors, nurses and laboratory staff).
- Patients requiring repeated transfusions (including haemophiliacs).
- Renal dialysis patients.
- Staff and patients in institutions looking after those with severe learning difficulties.
- Those who intend residing in highly endemic areas.
- Those accidentally exposed to HBsAg-positive blood.

Vaccination is unnecessary for those with a positive HBsAb or HBcAb.

People >50 years old, HIV-positive patients, those with concomitant diseases and 5–10% of healthy individuals have a poor or absent antibody response. Some may respond to a booster.

Immunization takes up to 12 months to confer adequate protection. This can be assessed by monitoring serum HBsAb levels. The duration of protection is not known but a single booster 5 years after the primary course is recommended, and may provide lifelong immunity.

Screening for hepatocellular carcinoma

Chronic carriers of HBsAg have a 100-fold increased risk of developing hepatocellular carcinoma. Those at greatest risk are males over 45 years old. This group should be screened at 6-monthly intervals with AFP levels and liver ultrasound examinations.

Hepatitis D (delta virus)

HDV (or delta virus) is a small RNA particle coated with HBsAg. It does not cause disease on its own and is only able to replicate when activated in the presence of HBV. It may either cause simultaneous infection with HBV (co-infection) or infect a chronic HBsAg carrier (superinfection). The risk factors for its transmission are the same as those for HBV infection;

however, HDV is particularly frequent in i.v. drug abusers. In addition, it may be spread by close personal contact and may be reactivated by HIV infection. It is present worldwide, but is rare in the UK.

Diagnosis	• Diagnosis is made by demonstrating anti-HDV antibodies with IgM HBcAb in the serum of a patient with chronic liver disease. IgM anti-HDV falls with resolution of infection. • Delta virus inhibits further HBV synthesis, so most patients do not have HBeAg and HBV DNA, and up to 10% are HBsAg negative. • Confirmation of the diagnosis is made by the detection of HDV DNA in serum and liver by PCR.
Clinical features	With co-infection, the clinical course is usually the same as that with hepatitis B alone, except that fulminant hepatitis is more frequent. A second rise in transaminases may occur after HDV superinfection. Delta virus superinfection should always be suspected in a stable HBsAg-positive patient who has a relapse.
Treatment	Treatment is generally unsatisfactory. High doses of interferon (e.g. 10 million units, three times a week) for prolonged periods (12 months) leads to sustained improvements in 15–25% of patients, but with a high incidence of adverse effects.
Prevention	At-risk individuals (see under Hepatitis B, above) should receive the HBV vaccine, which will also protect against HDV infection. Those who are already HBV carriers should be informed of the risks of acquiring HDV by continued i.v. drug use.

Further reading

Hoofnagle JH, Di Bisceglie AM. The treatment of chronic viral hepatitis. *New England Journal of Medicine*, 1997; **336**: 347–56.

Lee WM. Hepatitis B virus infection. *New England Journal of Medicine*, 1997; **337**: 1733–45.

Sherlock S, Dooley J. Viral hepatitis. In: *Diseases of the Liver and Biliary System,* 10th edn. Oxford: Blackwell Science, 1997; 265–302.

Related topics of interest

HEPATITIS C, E AND G

Hepatitis C

HCV, an RNA virus, is the commonest cause of post-transfusion and community-acquired non-A, non-B hepatitis and cryptogenic cirrhosis. There are an estimated 300 million carriers worldwide – 1.4% of the US population and up to 4–6% of those living in parts of Africa and the Middle East.

Different genotypes exist which differ in their disease severity and treatment response. The commonest subtypes in the Western world are types 1a and 1b, the latter being associated with more advanced disease and resistance to standard treatments. HCV is transmitted predominantly through contaminated blood and less effectively through infected bodily secretions (saliva, urine, semen). It is much less infectious than HBV.

At-risk groups include:

- Intravenous drug users (the commonest single cause, and associated with a >70% prevalence of infection).
- Haemophiliacs or others receiving blood products (ELISA screening is now virtually 100% effective at preventing transmission).
- Sexually active homosexuals.
- Those with multiple sexual partners.
- Organ transplant recipients.
- Renal dialysis patients.
- Those with tattoos.
- Babies born to infected mothers (usually only in the setting of high viral load or concomitant HIV infection).

Seroconversion after a needlestick injury from an index case infected with HCV ranges from 0–10%. Dentists and surgeons (particularly oral surgeons) are at risk of acquiring HCV, and infected surgeons may transmit the virus to their patients.

In up to half of patients, the mode of transmission is unknown.

Diagnosis	• ELISA-detected antibodies to HCV (anti-HCV) is the screening test of choice. Third-generation RIBA assays are more accurate and are used to confirm the result. Antibodies are detectable 6–8 weeks after infection and remain positive for life.
	• Detection of HCV RNA by PCR implies infectivity (rather than simply previous exposure). The test is used to confirm the ELISA test if it is equivocal and to monitor the response to treatment.
	• Serum transaminase levels fluctuate and correlate poorly with disease activity.
	• Disease activity and treatment options are best assessed on histological findings obtained by liver biopsy.
Clinical manifestations	The incubation period is 15–150 days. The symptoms are milder than for other causes of viral hepatitis; most patients

are asymptomatic and only a quarter of post-transfusion hepatitis cases develop jaundice. Some patients present with advanced chronic liver disease and its complications. Eighty percent of cases develop chronic hepatitis, and an estimated 30% develop cirrhosis and liver carcinoma within 30–40 years.

Associations with HCV infection include type II cryoglobulinaemia, membranoproliferative glomerulonephritis, porphyria cutanea tarda, thyroiditis and positive autoantibody titres (e.g. rheumatoid factor, antinuclear antibody).

Treatment

Excessive alcohol may synergistically aggravate liver injury, but small amounts are permissible. Older patients with post-transfusion HCV infection will usually outlive the sequelae of chronic liver disease and should be reassured. The aim of treatment is the early eradication of HCV before permanent liver damage ensues. IFN-α, with or without ribavirin, is the most widely used treatment.

Factors predicting a favourable response to IFN-α are:

- Age <45 years.
- Duration of disease <5 years.
- Absence of cirrhosis.
- Low iron concentrations in liver tissue.
- Low levels of genetic diversity of HCV ('quasi-species').
- Low serum and liver HCV RNA titres.
- HCV genotypes 2 and 3.

The last two factors are the most important independent predictors of a favourable response.

Other proposed factors indicating a favourable response to IFN-α are female sex, absence of immunosuppression (e.g. HIV infection), non-obese, no co-infection with HBV, no excessive alcohol intake and minimally elevated liver enzymes.

All chronic carriers of HCV should be regularly screened for hepatocellular carcinoma with liver ultrasound examinations and AFP levels in the same way as chronic HBV carriers.

Hepatitis E

Hepatitis E virus (HEV) is an RNA virus that causes sporadic and large-scale epidemics of viral hepatitis in developing countries. It is spread through sewage-contaminated water. It is a common cause of non-A, non-B, non-C hepatitis in the Far East, and is usually only found in Western countries in travellers to developing areas.

Clinical features and diagnosis

In endemic areas, HEV infects mainly young adults, and the clinical course resembles HAV infection. The infection is self-limiting and chronic infection does not occur. It may cause fulminant hepatitis, particularly in women in the last trimester of pregnancy, when the mortality is about 25%. The diagnosis is made by the detection of anti-HEV IgM and IgG antibodies in serial serum samples.

Hepatitis G

The clinical significance of hepatitis G virus (HGV) is uncertain – it is unclear whether it is an incidental agent or a potentially serious pathogen. It is detected by the PCR method; no antibody test is currently available. One to two percent of blood donors test positive for HGV DNA, but this is likely to be an underestimate. It is more prevalent in those with HBV, HCV and HIV infection than the general population, and is likely to be transmitted in the same way as these viruses. Its role as a potential cause of non-A–E, community-acquired or post-transfusion hepatitis is likely to be minimal.

Further reading

Dusheiko GM, Khakoo S, Soni P, Grellier L. A rational approach to the management of hepatitis C infection. *British Medical Journal*, 1996; **312**: 357–64.

Hoofnagle JH, Di Bisceglie AM. The treatment of chronic viral hepatitis. *New England Journal of Medicine*, 1997; **336**: 347–56.

Miyakawa Y, Mayumi M. Hepatitis G virus – a true hepatitis virus or an accidental tourist? *New England Journal of Medicine*, 1997; **336**: 795–6.

Sharara AI, Hunt CM, Hamilton JD. Hepatitis C. *Annals of Internal Medicine*, 1996; **125**: 658–68.

Sherlock S, Dooley J. Viral hepatitis. In: *Diseases of the Liver and Biliary System*, 10th edn. Oxford: Blackwell Science, 1997; 265–302.

Related topics of interest

Abnormal liver tests (p. 1)
Cirrhosis (p. 40)
Hepatic tumours (p. 150)
Hepatitis B and D (p. 157)

HEREDITARY NEOPLASTIC SYNDROMES OF THE INTESTINE

Familial adenomatous polyposis

- Familial adenomatous polyposis (FAP) is an autosomal dominant condition resulting in the development of large numbers (typically >100) of adenomatous polyps in the large bowel.
- The disordered gene, termed the APC (adenomatous polyposis coli) gene, is located on the long arm of chromosome 5.
- The exact incidence of the disease is uncertain, but is estimated as 1 in 7000–16 000 live births.
- Untreated individuals develop colonic polyps from the late teens, which increase in number (usually in the thousands) and size, until symptoms (typically rectal bleeding) result in presentation in the third decade.
- Progression of the polyps to carcinoma is inevitable, and usually occurs in the fourth decade, suggesting a 10-year adenoma-to-carcinoma sequence (which is the same as for sporadic colorectal carcinomas).
- Untreated patients die at a mean age of 42 (the age range being considerable).

Extracolonic manifestations

A number of extracolonic manifestations occur and are also believed to be due to the single gene defect. They may present before the diagnosis of FAP is made, and their presence in a child should raise the suspicion of FAP. They include:

- Osteomas. These benign tumours may occur in any bone, but are most common in the mandible, where they are commonly associated with dental abnormalities.
- Epidermoid cysts. These benign lesions of the subcutaneous tissue occur most frequently on the scalp and face in those with FAP.
- Desmoid tumours. These are rare fibrous lesions of musculoaponeurotic soft tissue. In those with FAP, they are usually found in small bowel mesentery, rectus abdominus muscle or lararotomy scars. They are commoner in females and, although they are benign, they may invade locally and tend to recur after excision.
- Congenital hypertrophy of the retinal pigment epithelium. These are multiple areas of increased pigmentation found incidentally in the majority of patients.
- Gastro-duodenal polyps. These are being increasingly recognized as more patients are having therapeutic colectomies and are surviving longer.
  Fundal gland polyposis consists of small non-neoplastic areas of dilated glands in the fundus and is found in 80% of patients with FAP.

Gastric adenomas (usually in the antrum) occur in 2–13% of patients, and may rarely undergo malignant transformation. Adenomatous polyps of the duodenum, mainly peri-ampullary, are present in most patients. Malignant transformation is common, and carcinoma of the duodenum is an important cause of death in those with FAP.

- Miscellaneous tumours. Other less common tumours associated with FAP include small-bowel adenomas, benign and malignant tumours of the extrahepatic biliary tree, papillary carcinoma of the thyroid and medulloblastoma.

Treatment

Treatment is by prophylactic proctocolectomy. In those with extensive rectal polyps or with a low rectal carcinoma, the operation of choice is a panproctocolectomy with an ileostomy. Restorative proctocolectomy with ileal pouch and ileo–anal anastomosis is the ideal operation, but it is technically difficult and results in an increased stool frequency and occasionally incontinence, which may be unacceptable to some patients. Subtotal colectomy and ileorectal anastomosis is also commonly performed. This, however, requires 6-monthly follow-up sigmoidoscopies to detect recurrent rectal polyps, which occur in 10–60% of patients. Proctectomy should therefore be considered in middle age.

Screening

- The FAP Registry maintains a record of index cases and their families to facilitate the screening of relatives and surveillance of affected individuals.
- Screening by DNA analysis is possible but is still unreliable owing to the heterogeneity of the mutations at the locus. Prenatal testing of fetal DNA by chorionic villous sampling is possible if the parent wishes it.
- Screening of those at risk should begin in the late teens with a flexible sigmoidoscopy. If this is normal, screening should be continued 2-yearly until the age of 40. DNA analysis of family members may further help to stratify the risk in such cases.
- If initial screening shows polyposis, sigmoidoscopy should be repeated every 6–12 months, plus a full colonoscopy 2-yearly. The timing of surgery depends on the grade and number of polyps, and the wishes of the individual patient. Most colectomies are carried out in the late teens.
- Regular upper endoscopies should be performed in all affected patients to enable the early detection of gastro-duodenal cancers. There is no evidence, however, that this practice prevents cancer deaths.
- Screening for thyroid cancers in affected women should also be considered.

- The use of aspirin or sulindac has been show to inhibit the growth of colorectal polyps, and will possibly become standard treatment in the future. Although these agents may alter the phenotypic expression, they do not affect the underlying genetic mutation, therefore careful screening will still be required.

Peutz–Jeghers syndrome

- This is an autosomal dominant condition characterized by dark melanin pigmentation of the lips and buccal mucosa, and less commonly on the digits and peri-anal skin. The pigmentation is most prominent in childhood and may fade in later life.
- Hamartomatous polyps develop in the large and small bowel in 90%. Unlike FAP, few new polyps form after the age of 30, and some may regress.
- Small intestinal polyps may cause blood loss, intussusception or, rarely, infarction.
- Colonic polyps are less common, and rarely undergo neoplastic transformation, unlike the polyps in other areas of the gut. The risk for this is, however, not as high as for FAP.
- An increased risk of cancer in the uterus, ovary, testis, pancreas, liver, breast, lung and thyroid is also recognized.
- Management involves regular screening for the above cancers, as well as regular endoscopies/enteroscopies, small-bowel barium studies and colonoscopies. Larger polyps can be removed in some cases by therapeutic enteroscopy.
- Genetic markers for the disease are not yet available, but relatives should be assessed for the dermatological manifestations (which almost invariably occur) and, if present, the necessary screening investigations should be undertaken.

Juvenile polyposis

- This is an inherited condition in which multiple juvenile polyps (see 'Colonic polyps' (p. 52)) form in the colon, and to a lesser extent the stomach and small intestine.
- Most patients present within the first decade with rectal bleeding, diarrhoea, intussusception or protein-losing enteropathy.
- Associated conditions include macrocephaly, congenital heart disease, Meckel's diverticulum and gut malrotation.
- There is a small but significant increased risk of gastrointestinal cancers and, to a lesser extent, cancers elsewhere.
- Endoscopic surveillence and polypectomy is advisable.

Further reading

Calam J, Williamson RCI. Neoplastic and miscellaneous diseases of the small intestine. In: Misiewicz JJ, Pounder RE, Venables CW (eds). *Disease of the Gut and Pancreas*. Oxford: Blackwell Scientific Ltd, 1994; 649–76.

Related topics of interest

Colonic polyps (p. 52)   Colorectal cancer and screening (p. 55)

HIV INFECTION AND THE GUT

Mouth

Most patients with HIV will develop oral lesions.

Oral candidosis

This is common as part of the acute HIV syndrome; its incidence increases as the CD4 count falls. Several distinct clinical forms are described:

- Pseudomembranous (thrush) – removable white mucosal plaques.
- Erythematous – smooth red areas on the palate or dorsum of the tongue, which are frequently overlooked.
- Hyperplastic – non-removable white plaques (rare, and often misdiagnosed as oral hairy leucoplakia).
- Angular cheilitis – redness and fissuring in the corners of the mouth.

Treatment is with amphotericin, nystatin or clotrimazole oral lozenges; or once-daily oral fluconazole, ketoconazole or itraconazole tablets. Prophylactic treatment with one of the oral agents is an option for those with recurrent relapses.

Oral hairy leucoplakia

This presents as a white patch, usually on the lateral surface of the tongue, but it can be found anywhere on the oral mucosa. Incidence increases as the CD4 count falls, and heralds a more rapid progression to AIDS. It is caused by the Epstein–Barr virus (EBV). Diagnosis is confirmed by histology. The lesions resolve with high-dose acyclovir or gancyclovir, but the response is often short lived.

Aphthous ulcers

These occur predominantly on the buccal mucosa, labial mucosa and the lateral aspect of the tongue, and are commonly severe and prolonged. Larger lesions (>1 cm) may resemble herpetic or malignant ulcers, and should be biopsied. Topical steroids are the treatment of first choice; persistent larger ulcers often respond to thalidomide.

Periodontal disease

Linear gingival erythema (formerly 'HIV-gingivitis') is a painful red band at the gingival margin. Necrotizing ulcerative periodontitis (formerly 'HIV-periodontitis') is more severe and relatively common in the late stages of HIV disease. This causes painful destruction of periodontal tissue and loosening of the teeth. Smoking is an exacerbating factor. Treatment is with local debridement, irrigation with povidone-iodine, chlorhexidine mouthwashes and oral antibiotics.

Other virus infections
- Herpes simplex virus (HSV) infection causes painful vesicles which rupture to form ulcers, and may occur on any mucosal surface. Acyclovir is the treatment of choice, and foscarnet is used for severe or resistant cases.
- Disseminated cytomegalovirus (CMV) infection may cause mouth ulcers. The diagnosis is made by the finding of characteristic histological and immunohistochemistry features on biopsy.
- Varicella-zoster infection involving the trigeminal nerve presents as painful oral and skin lesions, and is treated in the early stages with acyclovir.
- Oral warts due to papillomavirus infection are a relatively frequent finding, and can be removed surgically, but tend to recur.

Other oral lesions
- Salivary gland enlargement is due to CD8 lymphocyte infiltration. This often signifies a slower progression of disease. Symptoms (pain, xerostomia, cosmetic disturbance) are rare.
- The reddish/purple lesions of Kaposi's sarcoma (KS) are commonly found in the mouth, and may be the first manifestation of this condition. A biopsy will confirm the diagnosis and help to exclude other lesions (e.g. pyogenic granuloma, bacillary angiomatosis, haemangioma, pigmentation from ketoconazole or zidovudine use). Smaller lesions may be debulked surgically or injected with vinblastine or a sclerosant. Larger lesions may require radiotherapy.
- Non-Hodgkin's lymphoma (NHL) may appear as single or multiple ulcers or as a discrete swelling. Biopsies will confirm the diagnosis.

Oesophagus

- *Candida albicans* is the commonest oesophageal infection (50–75% of cases). It is rare in those with CD4 counts of >200/mm^3. It is often associated with oropharyngeal candidiasis.
- The commonest viral infection is CMV, usually occurring in the setting of disseminated CMV infection. Diffuse oesophagitis, single or multiple ulcerations (often at the oesophagogastric junction) or giant ulcers may develop.
- Idiopathic oesophageal ulceration is as common as CMV ulceration, and both are only found in those with a CD4 count of <100/mm^3.
- Other causes of oesophageal disease in patients with AIDS include:
    Infections (HSV, EBV, *Mycobacterium tuberculosis* and *M. avium, Cryptosporidium parvum* and *Pneumocystis carinii*).
    GORD (see p. 129).
    Pill-induced oesophagitis (azidothymidine (AZT) and dideoxycytosine (ddC) have been linked).
    NHL.
    KS.

| Diagnosis and treatment | • | A diagnostic trial of fluconazole is warranted. Most patients with candidiasis will respond within 3 days. Those that have not responded after a week of treatment should have an endoscopy. |

Diagnosis and treatment

- A diagnostic trial of fluconazole is warranted. Most patients with candidiasis will respond within 3 days. Those that have not responded after a week of treatment should have an endoscopy.
- Those with classic symptoms of GORD should be treated with a proton pump inhibitor.
- Endoscopy is the most useful test to assess oesophageal disease in patients with AIDS. In those who have not responded to an empirical trial of fluconazole, the most common finding is a viral or idiopathic ulcer. Biopsies for histological and immunohistochemistry analysis, and culture are valuable. Brushings for cytology specimens are useful to confirm *Candida* and HSV infection.
- Idiopathic ulcers usually respond well to oral prednisolone or thalidomide.
- CMV oesophagitis is treated with gancyclovir or foscarnet. The relapse rate of CMV oesophagitis is about 50%, but prophylactic therapy with gancyclovir is not recommended unless CMV retinitis is present. The main adverse effect of gancyclovir is pancytopenia, which may be treated with GM-CSF. Foscarnet can cause hypocalcaemia, hypophosphataemia and renal dysfunction.

Enterocolitis and diarrhoea

Diarrhoea occurs at some stage of HIV infection in 66% of patients in the West and in almost all patients in developing countries. The pathogenesis is complex, involving multiple aetiologies, varying with the stage of disease. An infectious cause will be found in 50–85% of cases.

Aetiology

1. *Protozoa*
- *Cryptosporidium parvum (20% of cases)*. The diarrhoea may be voluminous and associated with abdominal cramps and muscle wasting. Fever is usually absent. In those with a CD4 count of $>300/mm^3$ the infection may be cleared, but in others it becomes a chronic debilitating illness with frequent relapses and remissions. The diagnosis is made on an acid-fast stain of the stool or enteric or colonic biopsies.
- *Microsporidia* are small intracellular protozoa that account for between 30 and 50% of HIV-associated diarrhoea. The diagnosis is traditionally made by electron microscopic examination of small bowel biopsies, but light microscopy of biopsies, stool or intestinal aspirates are becoming more accurate.
- Other protozoal infections include *Entamoeba histolytica, Giardia lamblia* (which seldom causes severe symptoms or malabsorption), *Blastocystis hominis, Isospora belli, Cyclospora* spp. (which is also a common cause of diarrhoea in immunocompetent individuals).

2. *Viruses*
- CMV infection is the commonest cause of colitis in AIDS patients. It usually occurs in the setting of disseminated infection, and can also cause duodenal and ileal ulceration (and occasionally perforation). The commonest presentation is watery or bloody diarrhoea, abdominal pain, tenderness and a low-grade fever. Biopsies show large mononuclear cells containing inclusion bodies surrounded by a clear halo (the characteristic 'owl's eye' appearance). Immunoperoxidase and DNA staining will confirm the diagnosis.
- HSV infection of the rectum causes proctitis and ulceration, which can only be differentiated from CMV infection histologically.

3. *Bacteria*
- *Mycobacterium avium* complex (MAC) is the commonest systemic bacterial infection in HIV patients. It is usually associated with CD4 counts of <50/mm^3, and presents with diarrhoea, fever, anaemia, weight loss and night sweats. Acid-fast staining of colonic or small bowel biopsies reveal the organisms within foamy macrophages. A positive stool culture indicates colonization only. The histological findings resemble those of Whipple's disease, but the organism is not acid-fast in Whipple's disease.
- Other bacterial infections (e.g. *Salmonella* spp., *Shigella* spp., *Campylobacter jejuni*, *E. coli*) usually cause acute diarrhoea, often associated with a high fever. The diagnosis is made with stool and blood cultures. Relapses are common after successful treatment with antibiotics. Recent evidence suggests that chronic infection with such organisms may be a cause of diarrhoea in late-stage AIDS patients.
- A frequently overlooked pathogen is *Clostridium difficile*, which may not be associated with prior antibiotic usage.

4. *HIV enteropathy.* An HIV enteropathy (comprising villous atrophy, chronic mucosal inflammation and malabsorption) has been postulated by the discovery of lamina propria mononuclear cells containing HIV genetic material. Whether this is due to the direct or indirect effects of HIV infection, or the presence of an undiagnosed or unrecognized organism, is uncertain.

5. *Other causes*
- The fungus *Histoplasma capsulatum* can colonize the colon and produce diarrhoea, fever, weight loss and abdominal pain. The diagnosis is made by the finding of intracellular yeast-like organisms in Giemsa-stained colonic biopsy specimens.

- *Mycobacterium tuberculosis* may rarely cause diarrhoea.
- All patients with HIV disease are lactose intolerant and the consumption of milk or other dairy products may lead to diarrhoea.
- Didanosine may cause diarrhoea and, like pentamidine, may cause pancreatitis and malabsorption.
- KS commonly involves the gastrointestinal tract and may cause diarrhoea and, rarely, haemorrhage or bowel obstruction. Endoscopic biopsies may miss the lesions as they tend to lie deep in the submucosa.
- The gastrointestinal tract is the third commonest site of extranodal lymphomas (after CNS and bone).

Clinical evaluation

The following is a guideline to the diagnosis of chronic diarrhoea in a patient with HIV disease. In practice this is rarely straightforward, and in all cases an open mind should be kept, as multiple aetiologies are often responsible.

- A clinical history should be obtained to establish the disease stage, past gastrointestinal infections, diet, medications and recent travel or contacts. Malabsorption is associated with large-volume, irregular bowel motions, often with dehydration. Colitis is associated with more regular, smaller-volume stools, which are often blood-stained.
- Patients should be examined to detect fever, weight loss, dehydration and blood loss.
- Three stool specimens should be obtained and analysed for the presence of *Giardia*, *Cryptosporidia*, amoebae, *Isospora, Cyclospora*, *Salmonella*, *Campylobacter*, *Shigella* and *C. difficile* toxin. For those with a CD4 count of $<100/\text{mm}^3$, *Microsporidia* and acid-fast bacilli should be sought.
- A urine specimen should be obtained for *Entamoeba intestinalis* spores.
- Those with negative initial investigations, and those who show no improvement with treatment for an identified organism, should be assessed by sigmoidoscopy and gastroscopy with colonic and small bowel biopsies.

Treatment

The following is an overview of the current treatment regimens.

- *Cryptosporidium.* No agent is completely effective but high-dose paromamycin or azithromycin are used with some success.
- *Microsporidium.* Albendazole may be effective but is experimental.
- *Cyclospora* and *Isospora*. Trimethoprim-sulphamethoxazole is used.
- *Giardia lamblia* is treated with metronidazole.

- *Salmonella* spp., *Shigella* spp. and *Campylobacter* spp. are treated as per antibiotic sensitivities. Ciprofloxacin is usually effective.
- MAC is treated with clarithromycin, ethambutol and either clofazimine, amikacin, ciprofloxacin or rifabutin.
- *C. difficile* is treated with metronidazole or vancomycin.
- CMV. Gancyclovir and/or foscarnet are used.
- HSV. Acyclovir, orally or i.v., famcyclovir or foscarnet are used.

Other measures
- Nutritional supplements should be provided. Parenteral nutrition may be needed for cases of severe malabsorption.
- Antimotility agents (e.g. loperamide) increase transit time and reduce stool frequency.
- Codeine or morphine increase circular muscle contraction and anal sphincter tone.
- Cholestyramine binds bile salts and is useful for small bowel disease.
- Bulk-forming agents, such as methylcellulose and fibre, adsorb free water and are paradoxically beneficial in patients with mild symptoms.
- Octreotide (a somatostatin analogue), through its inhibitor effect on the gastrointestinal tract, is sometimes useful for refractory diarrhoea.
- Phenothiazines and NSAIDs are also occasionally used.

Hepatic parenchymal disease

- Nearly all patients with AIDS will develop abnormal hepatic histology (commonly steatosis). This is usually manifest by deranged liver enzymes in the presence of one or more disseminated opportunistic infections. The vast majority of patients have non-specific liver involvement together with extrahepatic disease, and therefore a liver biopsy is not usually indicated for patients with AIDS and elevated liver enzymes. Only patients with MAC, KS and CMV infection involving the liver have characteristic histological features which are able to be diagnosed with a liver biopsy.
- MAC involves the liver in up to 50% of patients with AIDS. Most patients present with a fever and elevated liver enzymes. A liver biopsy may show granulomas, but these are frequently missed and often poorly formed. As MAC is a disseminated infection, a higher diagnostic yield is obtained with blood cultures and a bone marrow biopsy.
- Incidental liver metastases of KS are not uncommon, and they rarely cause complications.
- CMV infection in the liver is common, but is only clinically relevant when it involves the biliary tree.
- Almost the same risk factors for HIV apply for hepatitis B and C. Co-infection is common and HIV accelerates the course of liver disease from viral hepatitis. Patients with HIV who are at risk for hepatitis B should be vaccinated, although this is often unsuccessful owing to the altered immunity.
- Both Hodgkin's and non-Hodgkin's lymphoma complicate HIV disease, and liver involvement is relatively common.

- With the multiple medications used, drug-induced hepatitis should always be considered. Trimethoprim-sulphamethoxazole, pentamidine, sulphadiazine, antifungals, didanosine and gancyclovir can all cause elevated liver enzymes. Nearly all antimycobacterial agents are hepatotoxic, and their withdrawal should be the first step in the work-up of any HIV patient with elevated liver enzymes.
- HSV and adenovirus can cause an acute hepatitis in patients with AIDS, which may be severe but both are treatable if detected early.
- Disseminated *Pneumocystis carinii*, *Microsporidia*, *Cryptococcus neoformans* and *Histoplasma capsulatum* may be all be isolated from the liver. They may all present as elevated liver enzymes, but seldom cause serious liver disease.

Biliary tract disease

- Cryptosporidiosis, CMV and microsporidiosis commonly infect the biliary tree in those with a CD4 count of <50/mm^3. Symptomatic patients present with symptoms of acalculous cholecystitis (i.e. right-upper quadrant pain, fever, markedly elevated ALP and minimally elevated aminotransferases and bilirubin). An ultrasound scan may show a thickened, dilated gall bladder, or it may be normal. A laparoscopic cholecystectomy should be considered.
- AIDS cholangiopathy presents with similar clinical features. An ERCP is confirmatory and shows features of papillary stenosis and intrahepatic sclerosing cholangitis. Treatment is with endoscopic sphincterotomy and antibiotics (ascending bacterial cholangitis is a significant problem). Cryptosporidiosis, CMV and local HIV infection are proposed aetiologies.

Pancreatic disease

- Acute or chronic pancreatitis may be caused by drugs (e.g. pentamidine, dideoxyinosine (ddI), and less often ddC and trimethoprim-sulphamethoxazole). Several disseminated infections often involve the pancreas (e.g. CMV, toxoplasmosis, *Cryptococcus*), but usually only cause asymptomatic amylasaemia, and rarely clinical acute pancreatitis.
- Circulating immune complexes may bind to amylase producing macroamylasaemia. This should be tested for, as it obviates the need for further investigations (e.g. ERCP).

Further reading

Blanshard C, Gazzard BG. Natural history and prognosis of diarrhoea of unknown cause in patients with acquired immunodeficiency syndrome (AIDS). *Gut*, 1995; **36**: 283–6.
Greenspan D, Greenspan JS. HIV-related oral disease. *Lancet*, 1996; **348**: 729–33.

Related topics of interest

IRRITABLE BOWEL SYNDROME

The irritable bowel syndrome (IBS) is probably the commonest condition encountered by gastroenterologists. It affects approximately 20% of adults in the western world, although less than a third consult a doctor. Men and women are affected equally but women are more likely to consult a doctor. The condition forms part of a large number of functional gastrointestinal disorders (i.e. those not explained by any structural or biochemical abnormality), and is characterized by abdominal discomfort (often minor) associated with defecation or a change in bowel habit, with the additional features of disordered defecation and abdominal distension.

The Rome diagnostic criteria

IBS is defined as at least 3 months of continuous or recurrent symptoms of:

(a) Abdominal pain/discomfort which is:
- Relieved with defecation and/or
- Associated with change in frequency or consistency of stool.

(b) Two or more of the following, on at least a quarter of occasions/days:
- More than three bowel movements/day or fewer than three bowel movements/week.
- Altered form of stool (lumpy/hard or loose/watery).
- Altered passage of stool (straining, urgency or sensation of incomplete evacuation).
- Passage of mucus.
- Bloating or feeling of abdominal distension.

Potential causes

1. Disordered gut motility. In patients with predominant constipation, some studies have shown that the colon is more sensitive to physiological stimuli (e.g. balloon distension, cholecystokinin) than healthy controls. Motility studies of the small bowel have shown clusters of contractions during fasting in some patients. Whole-bowel transit time is reduced in some patients with predominant diarrhoea. No disorder in motility has been consistently found and therefore no unifying hypothesis can be drawn from these studies.

2. Disorder of gut sensation. Several studies have shown an increased sensitivity to balloon distension of the rectum, colon and small bowel; these findings do not occur in the setting of a reduced pain threshold to other painful stimuli. It therefore seems possible that increased visceral sensation of the bowel plays some part in the cause of IBS.

3. Neurological. Disruption of central regulation of visceral sensation and motility may be more important than specific primary end-organ dysfunction. This is supported by the fact that symptoms involving the smooth muscle of the UGT, genitourinary system and bronchial tree are common in those with IBS.

4. Psychological factors. Psychological symptoms including depression, anxiety, phobia and somatization are more common in those with IBS than in healthy controls. Undoubtedly, psychological factors can alter the function of the gut, and several studies have shown that an episode of social stress often precedes the onset of symptoms. Those with IBS who consult a doctor seem to have a different attitude to illness in general compared to those who do not present, and this may be due to an underlying, poorly understood mood disorder.

5. Post-dysenteric IBS. Some patients with no prior affective disorder develop IBS following an episode of traveller's diarrhoea or food poisoning ('post-dysenteric IBS'). Although post-dysenteric IBS remains largely anecdotal, it is possible that certain external infective factors may trigger a chronic somatic dysfunction in a small number of patients.

6. Malabsorption of bile salts. This may be a factor in some patients, particularly if diarrhoea is predominant.

7. Food intolerance. A proportion of patients (particularly those with predominant gas and bloating) respond to trials of exclusion of wheat, dairy products or other dietary elements.

Investigations

The first step is to exclude organic disease with the minimum of appropriate investigations (i.e. do not over-investigate). Factors which would make one exclude organic disease more rigorously include:

- Age >45 years.
- Symptoms <6 months.
- Weight loss/anorexia.
- Rectal bleeding.
- Mouth ulcers.
- Arthralgias.
- Family history of polyps/colorectal carcinoma.
- Nocturnal diarrhoea.
- Progressively worsening constipation and/or diarrhoea (patients who alternate between constipation and diarrhoea usually have a functional cause).

A full blood count, urea, electrolytes, liver enzymes, thyroid function tests, ESR and CRP should be checked in all cases. A sigmoidoscopy and rectal biopsy should be performed to exclude inflammation and melanosis coli, especially in patients with diarrhoea-predominant IBS. A stool culture should be sent if diarrhoea is present. Further investigations (e.g. endoscopy, colonoscopy, barium enema, biliary and pancreatic ultrasound, small-bowel barium studies) should be guided by the predominant symptoms. In the average young patient, however, with a long history of typical symptoms with normal blood tests and rectal biopsy, further investigation is likely to be unrewarding and a positive diagnosis of IBS should be made.

Treatment

Time should be taken to explain carefully and sympathetically the possible mechanisms of symptom production and to reassure the patient of the lack of serious underlying disease (many patients being concerned that they may have cancer). Patients should be made aware that symptoms usually resolve (perhaps after months or years) and that, although there is no cure, symptoms can be relieved. Between 40 and 70% of patients respond to placebo.

1. Dietary modification. Although no specific diet helps all patients, almost half of patients experience some relief with an exclusion diet consisting of one meat, one source of carbohydrate and one fruit. Such patients are able to identify several agents (most commonly sorbitol, caffeine or wheat products) which exacerbate the symptoms when reintroduced into the diet. A small subgroup of patients have a defined food sensitivity, usually lactose intolerance. Such patients should withhold dairy products as a therapeutic trial. A high-fibre diet is useful in those with predominant constipation (it is cheaper than Fybogel); however, supplementing bran to the diet is not usually beneficial and may make flatulence, bloating and diarrhoea worse. Other dietary manipulation for those with constipation includes an increased intake of wholemeal rice/pasta, boiled vegetables and fluids (while being aware that some will worsen with increased wheat product intake, and require synthetic bulking agents (e.g. Fybogel) as a trial instead).

Those with predominant diarrhoea or abdominal pain should reduce dietary fat, tea and coffee. Stopping smoking may benefit some patients with diarrhoea. Patients with predominant gastric bloating may benefit from lactose and wheat avoidance.

2. End-organ treatment
- Medical therapy can be useful for the short-term amelioration of symptoms, although many patients would prefer to manage without. It is often necessary to try several different preparations, as the response may be unpredictable and vary with time, possibly due to a high placebo response rate in patients with IBS.
- Some patients with bowel frequency may benefit from an antidiarrhoeal agent (e.g. loperamide, up to 12 mg/day).

Codeine preparations are best avoided due to the risk of dependancy with long-term use.

- Constipation is best treated with dietary manipulation and/or laxatives (bulk forming, e.g. natural fibre/Fybogel; stool softening, e.g. sodium docusate; or osmotic, e.g. magnesium hydroxide).
- Abdominal pain may be relieved with antispasmodics (e.g. mebeverine, 135 mg three times daily; alverine subcitrate, 60 mg three times daily) or antimuscarinics (e.g. buscopan, 10 mg three times daily). For those with predominant constipation and bloating, peppermint oil (colpermin, one to two capsules three times daily) is preferable. It may worsen dyspepsia in susceptible patients, however.
- Prokinetic agents (e.g. domperidone, 10–20 mg three times daily before food; cisapride, 10 mg three times daily) may help patients with bloating, nausea and belching.

3. Central treatment. An underlying affective disorder may or may not be the cause of IBS; however, it is often a reason why a patient seeks medical advice. Psychotherapy and hypnosis (and to a lesser extent, antidepressants) do benefit those with severe symptoms. Although antidepressants do not work in non-depressed patients, they do alter small-bowel motility (imipramine slows intestinal transit whereas paroxetine accelerates motility). Tricyclics may therefore be useful for those with predominant diarrhoea, while serotonin reuptake inhibitors may be used for those with predominant constipation.

Further reading

Farthing MJG. Irritable bowel, irritable body, or irritable brain? *British Medical Journal,* 1995; **310:** 171–5.
Maxwell PR, Mendall MA, Kumar D. Irritable bowel syndrome. *Lancet,* 1997; **350:** 1691–4.
Spiller RC, Creed F. Irritable bowel or irritable mind? *British Medical Journal,* 1994; **309:** 1646–8.

Related topic of interest

Oesophageal dysmotility (p. 219)

JAUNDICE

Classification of jaundice The causes of jaundice may be classified into three broad categories. In practice, however, hepatic and cholestatic causes frequently coexist.

1. Prehepatic. This is usually Gilbert's disease or haemolysis (e.g. due to hereditary spherocytosis, sickle cell disease). It is characterized by an unconjugated hyperbilirubinaemia, normal liver enzymes and absent urinary bilirubin.

2. Hepatic
- Hepatitis – viruses, alcohol, drugs, other infections (e.g. Weil's disease).
- Cirrhosis – as above, plus primary biliary cirrhosis, metabolic (e.g. Wilson's disease, haemochromatosis).
- Other – Budd–Chiari syndrome, right heart failure, liver diseases of pregnancy, Dubin–Johnson syndrome.

These are usually characterized by mixed conjugated and unconjugated hyperbilirubinaemia with raised liver aminotransferases. Features of hepatocellular failure may be evident.

3. Cholestatic. Cholestatic (or obstructive) jaundice may be due to an obstruction at any level in the biliary system, and is classified according to whether the extrahepatic and larger intrahepatic ducts are dilated (extrahepatic cholestasis) or non-dilated (intrahepatic cholestasis).

(a) Causes of intrahepatic cholestasis (non-dilated ducts)
- Hepatitis – viral, alcoholic.
- Cirrhosis – any cause.
- Primary sclerosing cholangitis (PSC).
- Extensive metastases.
- Septicaemia.
- Drugs (e.g. antibiotics, phenothiazines, sex hormones).

(b) Causes of extrahepatic cholestasis (dilated ducts)
- Common bile duct stones.
- Carcinoma of the head of pancreas.
- Lymphadenopathy in porta hepatis.
- Pancreatitis (acute, chronic).
- Postsurgery or ERCP stricture.
- Cholangiocarcinoma.
- Choledochal cyst.
- Pancreatic pseudocyst.

Characteristically, a conjugated hyperbilirubinaemia and elevated ALP and GGT are found. Malabsorption may be evident (indicated by steatorrhoea, reduced calcium and vitamins A, D, E and K).

Diagnostic approach to jaundice

1. *History*
(a) Age. Younger patients are more likely to have a viral hepatitis (there are few clinical signs; may have enlarged, tender liver and splenomegaly) or a drug-induced cause, whilst in the elderly, mechanical obstructing lesions (gallstones, malignancy) are more common.
(b) Onset
- Rapid onset preceded by nausea, anorexia and aversion to smoking (hepatitis A or drug hepatitis).
- Slow onset with pruritus and few other symptoms (cholestatic jaundice).
- Persistent or episodic mild jaundice (haemolysis, familial hyperbilirubinaemias).
(c) Occupation
- Alcohol.
- Exposure to rats (leptospirosis).
- Industrial exposure.
(d) Travel
- Hepatitis endemic areas.
- Vaccinations received.
(e) Family history
- Haemolytic anaemias.
- Autoimmune diseases.
- Inflammatory bowel disease.
- Congenital hyperbilirubinaemias.
- Gallstones.
(f) Drugs
- Prescribed.
- Illicit.
- 'Alternative'.
- Intravenous.
(g) Contacts
- Sexual contacts.
- Blood transfusions.
- Close contacts at work or home.
- Tattoos.
- Dental work.
- Food (shellfish or unwashed foods).
(h) Medical history
- Operations (including biliary surgery or ERCP).
- Gallstones.
- Blood or clotting factor transfusions.
- Previous carcinomas (metastases).

(i) Associated symptoms
- Symptoms of underlying carcinoma.
- Pale stool and dark urine (cholestatic and sometimes hepatic jaundice).
- Pain (acute – pancreatitis, gallstones; chronic – pancreatic carcinoma, metastases, alcoholic hepatitis).
- Fever and rigors (cholangitis).

2. *Examination*
(a) Chronic liver disease
- Purpura.
- Bruising.
- Palmar erythema.
- Leuconychia.
- Muscle wasting.
- Clubbing.
- Dupuytren's contracture.
- Spider naevi.
- Oedema.
- Ascites.
- Splenomegaly.
- Loss of axillary/pubic hair.
- Testicular atrophy.

(b) Cholestasis
- Scratch marks.
- Polished nails from itching.
- Clubbing.
- Xanthelasmas.
- Xanthomas.
- Hepatomegaly.

(c) Hepatic encephalopathy
- Foetor.
- Asterixis.
- Confusion.

(d) Portal hypertension
- Ascites.
- Splenomegaly.
- Caput medusae (dilated veins radiating away from the umbilicus, as compared with inferior vena cava obstruction, where the flow is towards the head).

(e) Other signs
- Ulcers and pigmentation of the shins (chronic haemolysis).
- Ascites and large, nodular liver (carcinoma – primary or secondary).
- Smooth, enlarged liver (alcoholic liver disease, haemolysis, cholestasis, right heart failure).

- Arterial bruit (hepatoma or acute alcoholic hepatitis).
- Palpable gall bladder (pancreatic carcinoma).

3. *Investigations*

(a) Laboratory tests

- Bilirubin – confirms jaundice; the highest levels are found in cholestatic jaundice and the lowest in prehepatic jaundice.
- Liver enzymes – aminotransferases are highest in hepatocellular jaundice and normal in prehepatic jaundice.

    ALP – more than three times elevated (in the absence of bone disease, particularly Paget's disease) strongly suggests cholestasis. It is usually also elevated in hepatocellular jaundice in a similar magnitude to aminotransferases.

    GGT – elevated in cholestatic jaundice and also hepatocellular jaundice. A change in the level rather than the absolute level is indicative of alcohol consumption.
- Prothrombin time and albumin. These are both indicators of hepatic synthetic function and are therefore abnormal in acute or chronic liver failure. Albumin is depressed in any cause of chronic liver disease (usually with elevated globulin levels). PT is correctable with vitamin K in cholestatic jaundice but not in hepatocellular jaundice.
- Leucocyte count. This is low with relative lymphocytosis in hepatocellular jaundice, and high with polymorph predominance in viral hepatitis, alcoholic hepatitis and cholangitis. It is also raised in carcinoma (primary or secondary).
- Urine tests. Bilirubinuria is present in hepatic jaundice and absent in prehepatic causes. Urobilinogen is present in haemolytic jaundice and absent in complete cholestasis.
- Stool. A pale (acholic) stool indicates cholestasis. Rectal bleeding (occult or overt) indicates malignancy or bleeding from varices.

(b) Radiology

- Chest radiograph – primary or secondary lung carcinoma.
- Abdominal ultrasound. This distinguishes obstructive jaundice (dilated bile ducts) from non-obstructive jaundice. The cause of obstruction may be evident, e.g. gallstones, hepatic metastases, lymphadenopathy in the porta hepatis or carcinoma of the pancreatic head. Signs of portal hypertension (splenomegaly, ascites, portal and splenic vein blood flow) and hepatic vein patency (Budd–Chiari syndrome) also can be assessed.

4. *Further investigations.* Once the type of jaundice has been established, subsequent tests are aimed at determining the exact cause.

(a) Prehepatic jaundice

- Gilbert's disease is the commost cause of mild unconjugated hyperbilirubinaemia. Other enzymes should be normal and haemolysis excluded. Bilirubin rises with fasting, but this is not specific for Gilbert's disease. A family history (autosomal dominant) is helpful.
- Haemolysis is sought with a reticulocyte count, Coomb's test and serum haptoglobin (low in haemolysis). Other tests might include erythrocyte fragility test (hereditary spherocytosis), Ham's acid lysis test (paroxysmal nocturnal haemoglobinuria), haemoglobin electrophoresis (sickle cell disease) and a bone marrow biopsy.

(b) Hepatic jaundice

- Acute

  Viral serology (hepatitis A, B, D, E, Epstein–Barr virus (EBV), Dengue fever, cytomegalovirus (CMV), herpes simplex, flavivirus (yellow fever), arenavirus (Lassa fever)).

  Leptospira, *Mycoplasma*, *Rickettsia* serology.

  Blood alcohol levels, drug levels (e.g. paracetamol, antituberculous and antiepileptic drugs).

- Chronic

  Hepatitis B and C serology.

  Anti-smooth muscle, anti-nuclear and anti-LKM antibodies (autoimmune hepatitis).

  AMA (PBC).

  Serum iron, ferritin, iron binding capacity (haemochromatosis), serum copper, caeruloplasmin, 24-hour urinary copper (Wilson's disease).

Percutaneous liver biopsy is often useful to assess causes of chronic hepatic jaundice, but is rarely needed in acute jaundice. An ultrasound-guided approach is safest and is used to target the biopsy to a specific lesion. The transjugular approach is used in the presence of a clotting disorder.

(c) Cholestatic/obstructive jaundice

- ERCP is the investigation of choice if the cause has not been established by ultrasound. Small common bile duct stones may be missed on ultrasound and they may cause intermittant obstruction. It is also used to confirm primary sclerosing cholangitis and malignant strictures (cholangiocarcinomas, ampullary tumours and carcinoma of the head of the pancreas) with the aid of biopsies and brushings. ERCP is also used therapeutically to remove common bile duct stones, perform a sphincterotomy and place biliary stents.

  An obstructing lesion demonstrated by ultrasound or

ERCP is further assessed with a CT scan, possibly with a guided biopsy.

- PTC can be used in the small number of patients in whom ERCP is technically impossible.
- Magnetic resonance cholangiography (MRC) is a non-invasive method of imaging the biliary tree, and may obviate the need for diagnostic ERCP in certain patients in the future.

Familial hyperbilirubinaemias

Gilbert's syndrome

- This common, probably autosomal dominant condition affects about 2% of the population.
- A deficiency in bilirubin glucuronidase produces an unconjugated hyperbilirubinaemia, which is usually detected by chance on routine screening.
- The jaundice is mild and may be noticeable with fasting, during an intercurrent illness or after drinking alcohol.
- There are no other abnormal physical signs.
- Bilirubin levels of 17–85 μmol/l are usual (conjugated bilirubin levels are normal), and liver enzymes, tests for haemolysis and hepatic histology (not routinely required) are normal.
- Patients have a normal life expectancy, and no treatment other than reassurance is necessary.

Crigler–Najjar syndrome

1. Type-I. This is an autosomal recessive condition resulting in the absence of glucuronyl transferase and severe unconjugated hyperbilirubinaemia. Most patients die due to kernicterus in the first year of life. Phototherapy is temporarily effective and liver transplantation is curative.

2. Type-II. Glucuronyl transferase levels are markedly reduced, unconjugated bilirubin levels are very high, but patients are able to survive into adulthood. Phenobarbitone, and occasionally phototherapy, are standard treatments.

Dubin–Johnson syndrome

- This benign, autosomal recessive condition results in a conjugated hyperbilirubinaemia due to defective excretion of bile into the canaliculi.
- Jaundice is mild and intermittent and may occur during pregnancy or after taking oral contraceptives.
- The liver is macroscopically greenish black (the nature of the pigment is uncertain), but the architecture is normal.
- Liver enzymes are not elevated.
- A late rise in the prolonged bromsulphthalein (BSP) test is characteristic.

- Intravenous cholangiography shows no uptake in the biliary system.
- The prognosis is excellent.

Rotor syndrome Like the Dubin–Johnson syndrome, this is a familial conjugated hyperbilirubinaemia with an excellent prognosis. It differs from Dubin–Johnson syndrome in that there is no abnormal liver pigmentation, no late rise in the BSP test and the i.v. cholangiogram is normal.

Further reading

Berk PD, Noyer C. Bilirubin metabolism and the hereditary hyperbilirubinaemias. *Seminars in Liver Disease*, 1994; **14**: 323.

Frank BB. Clinical evaluation of jaundice. A guideline of the patient care committee of the American Gastroenterological Association. *Journal of the American Medical Association*, 1989; **262**: 3031.

Related topic of interest

Abnormal liver tests (p. 1)

LIVER DISEASE IN PREGNANCY

Normal pregnancy results in mild, benign cholestasis. ALP levels are moderately elevated (mostly of placental origin), but bilirubin, transaminase and GGT levels are normal. Jaundice in pregnancy is either due to a condition unique to pregnancy (as discussed here) or is caused by an intercurrent process (e.g. gallstones or viral hepatitis).

Acute fatty liver of pregnancy

This rare condition occurs only in the third trimester and presents as nausea, recurrent vomiting and abdominal pain (in 50%) followed by jaundice. Other clinical features include oedema, ascites, hypertension and proteinuria. Severe cases progress to coma, renal failure and DIC, with death being due to extensive haemorrhage. It is commoner in pregnancy with twins and in primigravidae, and usually does not recur in subsequent pregnancies. The condition is caused by a systemic defect in mitochondrial function and forms part of the 'mitochondrial cytopathies' (comprising acute fatty liver of pregnancy, Reye's syndrome and genetic defects of mitochondrial function).

Biochemical tests reveal elevated ammonia, uric acid and transaminase levels, hypoglycaemia and, as with other mitochondrial cytopathies, lactic acidosis. Jaundice is invariable (as compared with toxaemias of pregnancy) and occurs in the absence of haemolysis. Leucocytosis, thrombocytopenia and deranged clotting are common, and DIC occurs in 10%.

A liver biopsy is not necessary for the diagnosis, but will show enlarged, foamy hepatocytes containing fat droplets, with minimal surrounding inflammation.

Management of mild cases involves hospital admission for close monitoring of clinical and laboratory features. The pregnancy should be terminated if there is any deterioration. Continued monitoring postpartum is important. Hypoglycaemia and coagulopathy should be corrected, renal function supported if it is deteriorating, and prophylaxis for gastrointestinal haemorrhage with a proton pump inhibitor or sucralfate given.

The condition was once almost invariably fatal; however, improved screening and early treatment of milder cases has dropped the fetal and maternal mortality to 0–20%.

Toxaemias of pregnancy

This comprises a spectrum of diseases which frequently overlap with acute fatty liver of pregnancy. Hypertension, fluid retention and proteinuria are characteristic. The aetiology is unknown but is thought to be related to an increased vascular sensitivity to endogenous pressor agents. The resultant endothelial damage, deranged clotting and arteriolar constriction predominantly affect the uterus, kidneys, liver and brain. Two recognized variants are pre-eclampsia and the HELLP syndrome (haemolysis, elevated liver enzymes, low platelet count). The two forms frequently overlap.

Mild cases of pre-eclampsia result in elevated ALP and transaminase levels, and thrombocytopenia, suggestive of early DIC. Severe cases present with epigastric pain (more commonly than with acute fatty liver), vomiting and hypertension, and markedly elevated liver enzymes. Unlike acute fatty liver, jaundice (and liver failure) is a late feature and is usually associated with DIC and a poor prognosis. Liver histology shows fibrin deposition, haemorrhages and later infarcts, with no inflammatory infiltrate. Pre-eclampsia complicated by DIC may result in hepatic infarction, haemorrhage or rupture. This is evident by the sudden onset of right-upper quadrant pain and hypovolaemic shock. The diagnosis is confirmed with an ultrasound or CT scan. Treatment is supportive for subcapsular haemorrhage (radiological embolization is an option), or surgical in severe cases. The pregnancy should be terminated in severe cases.

The HELLP syndrome often occurs with a background of previously uncomplicated pregnancies. Hypertension and proteinuria may be absent. The perinatal mortality is 10–60% and the maternal mortality is 1.5–5%.

Cholestasis of pregnancy

Cholestasis of pregnancy is an exaggeration of the normal physiological cholestasis which occurs in the third trimester of all pregnancies. It is often familial and is commonest in northern Europe, Chile and China. It is manifest by generalized pruritus, dark urine, pale stools and mild jaundice in an otherwise well patient. Pruritus may be mild, but is often the most distressing symptom. The symptoms resolve 1–2 weeks after delivery and tend to recur in subsequent pregnancies at varying times (usually earlier) and with increasing intensities. The aetiology is unknown, but it is possibly due to an increased sensitivity of canalicular cell membranes to oestrogens. Patients also commonly experience a similar illness if given oral contraceptives.

Investigations show an elevated conjugated bilirubin, ALP and prolonged PT. Liver aminotransferases are also usually elevated. Viral hepatitis, obstructive jaundice and PBC should be excluded.

Pruritus is treated with cholestyramine or ursodeoxycholic acid. All patients should be given vitamin K supplements to prevent postpartum haemorrhage. The prognosis for the mother is excellent; however, in severe cases, the fetus is at risk of prematurity and death. Close monitoring of the fetus is therefore needed, and the pregnancy terminated if fetal distress occurs.

Further reading

Reyes H, Sandoval L, Wainstein A *et al.* Acute fatty liver of pregnancy: a clinical study of 12 episodes in 11 patients. *Gut*, 1994; **35**: 101.
Riely CA. Hepatic disease in pregnancy. *American Journal of Medicine*, 1994; **96**: 117–85.

Related topics of interest

MALABSORPTION

Malabsorption occurs when one or more of the three phases of digestion and intestinal absorption is impaired.

The luminal phase

- This phase involves hydrolysis and solubilization of dietary protein, carbohydrate and fat, mainly by pancreatic and biliary secretions.
- Impairment of pancreatic lipase secretion results in fat malabsorption (steatorrhoea and fat-soluble vitamin deficiency). Causes include chronic pancreatitis, cystic fibrosis, carcinoma of the pancreas, and the Zollinger–Ellison syndrome (lipases inactivated by excess gastric acid).
- Fat malabsorption also occurs due to defects in the bile salt enterohepatic pathway. Causes include impaired:
    Production (parenchymal liver disease).
    Secretion (cholestatic jaundice, and impaired cholecystokinin release due to extensive mucosal disease (e.g. CD)).
    Deconjugation/binding (bacterial overgrowth).
    Conservation (terminal ileal resection/disease causing increased faecal loss of bile salts).

The mucosal phase

- This phase involves uptake and further hydrolysis of carbohydrates and peptides, and the packaging of fat by enterocytes.
- It is impaired by any cause of mucosal damage (e.g. CD, tropical sprue, Crohn's disease, radiation, ischaemia), resection (particularily ileal), and infiltrations (e.g. abetalipoproteinaemia, α-chain disease, small bowel lymphoma, amyloidosis).
- Drugs may also impair nutrient absorption at the mucosal level (e.g. colchicine, neomycin, methotrexate, mefenamic acid).

Removal phase

- This phase involves the transportation of absorbed nutrients into the lymph or portal blood.
- Lymphatic disease (e.g. primary intestinal lymphangiectasia) and possibly vascular insufficiency impair the removal phase.

Clinical assessment

History and examination
- Vague constitutional/gastrointestinal symptoms are common, and may be misinterpreted as IBS.
- Fat malabsorption is characterized by steatorrhoea (pale, bulky, malodorous stools that are difficult to flush away).

Pancreatic exocrine insufficiency is usually the cause when stools are oily, while mucosal small bowel disease is more likely when stools are more voluminous.

- Protein malabsorption produces weight loss and muscle wasting, peripheral oedema and leuconychia.
- Carbohydrate malabsorption leads to watery diarrhoea, abdominal distention, borborygmi, and excessive flatus.
- Weight loss is common in all cases and may be marked in some. It may, however, be minimal in cases of malabsorption of specific nutrients (e.g. vitamin B_{12} deficiency in ileal disease or bacterial overgrowth).
- Specific or multiple vitamin and mineral deficiencies are common in advanced cases. The clinical consequences of specific deficiencies are listed below:

  Iron: anaemia, koilonychia, cheilosis, glossitis, apht hous ulcers.

  Folic acid: anaemia, glossitis, aphthous ulcers.

  Vitamin B_{12}: anaemia, glossitis, neurological disorders.

  Vitamin A: xerophthalmia, night blindness, hyperkeratosis.

  Vitamin D: bone pain, osteomalacia, proximal myopathy.

  Vitamin E: neurological or psychological disturbance.

  Vitamin K: bleeding tendency.

  Calcium and magnesium: paraesthesias, tetany, muscle weakness.

  Zinc: anaemia, leucopenia, acrodermatitis, poor taste, poor wound healing.

- Abdominal pain may occur with chronic pancreatitis (epigastric, radiating to the back), subacute obstruction (intermittent, colicky, often accompanied by vomiting) or mesenteric ischaemia (postprandial, with food aversion).
- Certain systemic diseases may manifest with some features of malabsorption. These include thyroid disorders, Addison's disease, diabetes mellitus, systemic sclerosis and the vasculitides.
- A careful drug history should be obtained, as various antibiotics, antimetabolites and laxatives may induce malabsorption. Alcohol is a further frequently overlooked cause.
- Previous gastric or intestinal surgery may suggest a short bowel syndrome.

Investigations

1. *Initial blood tests*

- Full blood count and film, serum iron, vitamin B_{12} (reduced in terminal ileal disease and bacterial overgrowth) and red blood cell folate (commonly reduced in mucosal disease and may be elevated in bacterial over-growth) should be measured.

- Serum calcium and magnesium deficiency often coexists.
- ALP (an elevated level with a reduced calcium suggests osteomalacia) and albumin (if very low may suggest a protein-losing enteropathy, but is neither a sensitive nor specific test for malabsorption) should be measured.
- A prolonged PT, and low serum vitamin A, D and E levels can indicate fat-soluble vitamin malabsorption.

2. Tests to confirm malabsorption

(a) Tests of fat absorption. Fat absorption is dependent on the combined functions of the pancreas, biliary system and small bowel mucosa. Tests include:

- Sudan stain of a random faecal sample (not accurate in mild cases).
- Faecal fat estimation. This is the best method of detecting fat malabsorption but is unpopular. Stool markers should be used to estimate the completeness of collection. A 3-day faecal fat measurement is made whilst the patient is on a standardized diet (100 g fat per day begun 2 days prior to collection). An excretion of >6 g per day is abnormal.
- Carbon-14 (^{14}C)-triolein breath test. This is a radiolabelled triglyceride that, after absorption, releases radiolabelled CO_2 which is detectable in the breath. Low levels of $^{14}CO_2$ are found in fat malabsorption, but the test is inaccurate in those diseases causing abnormal triglyceride or CO_2 metabolism.

(b) Tests of carbohydrate absorption

- The lactose/hydrogen breath test. This involves ingestion of 50 g of lactose and the measurement of breath hydrogen. A rise of >20 ppm above the basal level indicates lactase deficiency. Those with normal lactase levels produce little or no breath hydrogen. False positives occur with small bowel bacterial overgrowth.
- A stool pH of <5.5 is suggestive, but not diagnostic, of carbohydrate malabsorption.

(c) Tests of protein absorption. Tests of protein absorption are seldom indicated in cases of malabsorption, except to confirm protein-losing enteropathy. Traditional tests are inconvenient and expensive. The ratio of the α_1-antitrypsin level in serum to that in a 24-hour stool specimen is a recently introduced and more practical alternative.

(d) Other tests

- The D-xylose excretion test is a sensitive test of small bowel mucosal integrity. After an overnight fast, 25 g of

D-xylose is ingested and urine collected for the next 5 hours. Less than 4 g of D-xylose in the urine collection is indicative of abnormal mucosal function. It is useful to establish the cause of steatorrhoea – a normal test suggests pancreatic exocrine insufficiency.

- The Schilling test helps to elicit the cause of vitamin B_{12} deficiency.
- The $[^{75}Se]$-homotaurocholic acid (SeHCAT) test is used to detect bile acid malabsorption in cases of steatorrhoea with no obvious ileal disease. In bile salt malabsorption, less than 5% of the SeHCAT is retained (compared to 80% retention in 24 hours and 19% retention at 7 days in healthy individuals).
- Therapeutic trials are often helpful, and may allow a rapid assessment of the likely problem, e.g. cholestyramine (for bile salt malabsorption); pancreatic supplements; antibiotics (for suspected small bowel overgrowth).

3. Identification of the site of malabsorption

- Multiple (at least four) low duodenal biopsies are needed to confirm coeliac disease and other causes of villous atrophy (see 'Coeliac disease' (p. 44)).
- To assess the jejunal mucosa, a small bowel (push) enteroscope may be used. Characteristic microscopic features are found in the following: Whipple's disease, lymphoma, abetalipoproteinaemia, amyloidosis, Crohn's disease, eosinophilic gastroenteritis, and certain infections (e.g. *Mycobacterium avium intracellulare* and *Cryptosporidia*). Measurement of enzyme levels in fresh mucosal biopsies are occasionally needed to detect disaccharidase deficiency.
- Duodenal juice microscopy may show *Giardia lamblia* or *Strongyloides stercoralis*.
- Small bowel radiology will usually identify jejunal diverticuli, stagnant loops, Crohn's disease, lymphoma and tumours.
- A CT scan of the abdomen may detect pancreatic or retroperitoneal lesions (e.g. lymphangiectasia).
- An explorative laparotomy may be needed if no diagnosis has been attained from the above tests.

4. Tests of exocrine pancreatic insufficiency. In many cases the diagnosis can be made on the clinical findings and routine investigations (including abdominal radiograph, abdominal ultrasound, ERCP). A number of tests are available to assess pancreatic function, but most are limited to specialist centres (details of protocols can be found in larger texts (see Further reading) or from the local chemical pathology service). Direct tests involve intubation of the duodenum and analysis of aspirated juice, e.g. the secretin test and the (less sensitive and specific) Lundh test meal. Indirect tests are done without oral intubation, and include the NBT-PABA test, the pancreolauryl test and the dual-label Schilling test (differential oral absorption of (i) ^{58}Co-labelled B_{12} bound to R protein, and (ii) ^{57}Co-labelled B_{12} bound to intrinsic factor: in pancreatic deficiency, urinary excretion ratio of ^{58}Co to ^{57}Co falls).

5. Tests of small bowel bacterial overgrowth. The diagnosis should be suspected in the postsurgical abdomen (where surgical blind loops and anastomoses between large and small bowel have been formed) and where strictures, fistulae and diverticulae exist (particularly in Crohn's disease).

- Bacterial counts of greater than 10^5 obtained via jejunal aspiration.
- The $[^{14}C]$glycocholic acid breath test (detects the ability of bacteria to deconjugate a radiolabelled bile salt). The test is positive if >4.5% of the administered radioactivity is released in the breath over 6 hours.
- The $[^{14}C]$D-xylose breath test works on similar principles and is possibly more accurate.
- The glucose/hydrogen breath test detects the rapid bacterial fermentation of a 50 g glucose load by measuring a breath hydrogen level >20 ppm compared to a fasting level. An early (<1 hour) breath hydrogen rise is typically seen in small bowel bacterial overgrowth.

Treatment

- Treatment is aimed at replacing the nutritional deficiencies and at correcting the underlying cause. For example, small bowel bacterial overgrowth is treated with antibiotics, pancreatic insufficiency with pancreatic supplements, and rapid gastric emptying after surgery with anticholinergics.
- Specific nutritional deficiencies should be corrected by enteral supplementation, and provision should be made for ongoing losses.
- Vitamin B_{12} supplements are needed after even limited ileal resection, while fat-soluble vitamins, calcium and magnesium are needed in cases of steatorrhoea and extensive small bowel resection.
- Dietary modification with a low-fat (30–50 g/day) and high-protein diet is usually only necessary if steatorrhoea is resistant to other treatment. Although steatorrhoea is improved, the total caloric intake may be suboptimal. In such cases, medium-chain triglycerides may be used as fat supplements to increase the caloric intake. They are more readily hydrolysed by pancreatic lipases, but are unpalatable and expensive.

- For those with extensive mucosal disease or intestinal resections, troublesome diarrhoea may be controlled with fat restriction. Those with predominantly ileal disease or resection may be helped with cholestyramine.

The consequences of malabsorption

Apart from the immediate problems of water and electrolyte losses and the long-term consequences of nutrient deficiencies, the following two manifestations should also be borne in mind in those patients with malabsorption.

- Hyperoxaluria occurs in those with bile salt malabsorption due to a paradoxical increased absorption from the gut. This may cause renal stones, and interstitial oxalate nephropathy in severe cases. Treatment is a low-oxalate diet (avoiding spinach, rhubarb, tea, cocoa and cola drinks). The condition occurs commonly in those with small-bowel Crohn's disease and in those with a jejuno-ileal bypass. Those with an ileostomy have a relatively increased water and bicarbonate loss from it, resulting in a concentrated, acidic urine, which predisposes to uric acid renal stones.
- Hyposplenism is particularly associated with coeliac disease, but is also found in tropical sprue, Whipple's disease and inflammatory bowel disease. This is recognized on the blood film by Howell–Jolly bodies and thrombocytopenia. It is also associated with a diminished primary antibody response, the clinical significance of which is uncertain.

Further reading

British Society of Gastroenterology. *Guidelines in Gastroenterology. Tests for Malabsorption*. London: British Society of Gastroenterology, September 1996.
Wetherall DJ, Leadingham JGC, and Warrell DA (eds). Malabsorption. In: *Oxford Textbook of Medicine*. Oxford: Oxford University Press, 1996; 1899–1935.

Related topics of interest

MALIGNANT TUMOURS OF THE STOMACH

Gastric carcinoma

Gastric cancer remains the second most common cause of cancer deaths worldwide. The incidence has been declining, particularly in western societies. The highest incidence is found in Japan (where it accounts for 20–30% of all cancers), China, South America and Eastern Europe. African Americans, Hispanic Americans and Native Americans have a 1.5–2.5 increased risk compared to white people in the USA. It is approximately twice as common in males than in females, is rare before the fifth decade and has a peak incidence in the seventh decade. Over 95% are adenocarcinomas; the remaining 5% being non-Hodgkin's lymphomas, leiomyosarcomas and, rarely, carcinoid tumours or squamous carcinomas.

Classification

Gastric adenocarcinoma may be divided into two histological categories: intestinal and diffuse. It is thought that they represent different aetiological entities, the intestinal type being more closely linked to environmental factors, and the diffuse type to genetic factors.

- The intestinal type probably arises from areas of intestinal metaplasia. It resembles colonic carcinoma histologically, is usually macroscopically discrete (ulcerated or polypoid) and usually occurs in the distal stomach. The intestinal type is commoner in areas with a high incidence of gastric carcinoma, and several environmental factors are thought to play a role. The overall incidence has fallen relative to the diffuse type.
- The diffuse type occurs more often in younger patients, and genetic rather than environmental factors are thought to be important. Macroscopically the tumour lacks a clear border and histologically it consists of infiltrating cells clumped in small numbers. Diffuse-type adenocarcinomas are generally associated with a poorer prognosis.

Approximately 50% of gastric carcinomas occur in the antral and prepyloric region, 20% on the lesser curve, 5% on the greater curve, 5% in the fundus, 10% in the cardia (although the relative incidence of the latter is increasing) and 10% are diffuse (linitus plastica or 'leather bottle stomach').

Predisposing factors

1. Medical conditions. Chronic atrophic gastritis, intestinal metaplasia, pernicious anaemia, Menetrier's disease (p. 201), gastric adenomatous polyps and partial gastrectomy are all thought to be precancerous conditions to variable degrees. Smokers have a two- to threefold increased risk of developing gastric cancer.

2. *H. pylori infection.* This is associated with a three- to six-fold increased risk compared to those without the organism. Benign gastric ulcers are thought not to be precancerous, although it should be remembered that malignant ulcers often closely resemble benign ulcers and may even partially regress with medical treatment.

3. *Nutritional factors and environmental factors.* Diets rich in salted, smoked, dried or preserved foods (i.e. nitrate rich) are associated with an increased risk, whereas those rich in fruit and vegetables have a reduced risk. The hypothesis is that certain intraluminal bacteria produce nitrate reductases, which convert dietary nitrates to nitrites which, in turn, interact with other dietary substrates to form nitrosamines. Such anaerobic bacteria are more often found in those with achlorhydria and atrophic gastritis. Nitrosamines are carcinogenic and induce dysplasia and eventually carcinoma *in situ*. The overall decreased incidence of the intestinal subtype is thought to be partly owing to improved methods of food preservation, enabling diets to be richer in fresh fruit and vegetables. It is also known that people and their offspring emigrating from areas of high risk to low-risk areas show a reduction in the risk of developing carcinoma, again suggesting important environmental factors.

4. *Socio-economic factors.* Overall, the risk of gastric cancer is inversely related to socio-economic status; however, the incidence of adenocarcinoma in the proximal stomach and gastro-oesophageal junction increases in those of higher socio-economic classes.

5. *Genetic influences.* First-degree relatives of an index patient have a two- to threefold increased risk. Those with FAP have an increased risk of upper gastrointestinal carcinomas. Furthermore, those with blood group A have an increased risk of developing the intestinal subtype. Mutations in the *p53* tumour suppressor gene are common in gastric carcinoma, and are associated with a decreased survival.

Clinical features

- Early gastric cancer is usually asymptomatic and when symptoms develop it is generally incurable. Even in advanced disease, there may be few physical signs.
- Possible early symptoms include non-specific upper abdominal discomfort (which may be indistinguishable from ulcer-type pain and is often relieved by antacids or H_2 blockers), weight loss, anorexia, nausea and, less frequently, melaena or haematemesis.
- Dysphagia may occur if the tumour is in the cardia, or vomiting if it is in the antrum, obstructing the pylorus.

- General examination may reveal cachexia, pallor, Virchow–Troissier node, Sister Joseph's nodule (periumbilical metastatic infiltration) or, rarely, dermatological features (metastatic nodules, acanthosis nigricans, Trousseau's sign (thrombophlebitis) or dermatomyositis).
- In advanced disease, an epigastric mass, hepatomegaly (liver metastasis), ascites (peritoneal metastasis) or a Krukenberg tumour (ovarian metastasis) may be detected.

Diagnostic investigations
- Endoscopy may reveal either an ulcer or a fungating polypoid lesion. Less than 3% of gastric ulcers are malignant and the diagnostic accuracy is greatly increased with obtaining six to eight biopsies from both the edge and, if possible, the base of the lesion. Adding brush cytology further improves diagnostic accuracy, and is particularly useful if the lesion is in an inaccessible position to biopsy.
- Diffusely infiltrating carcinomas may only be detected by a barium meal (showing a poorly distensible stomach). Endoscopic biopsies which extend to the submucosa will confirm the diagnosis in such cases.

Staging investigations
- Full blood count (which may show anaemia from blood loss, or a leucoerythroblastic picture in advanced disease), liver enzymes (a raised ALP and GGT suggest liver metastases, hypoalbuminaemia may be found due to an associated nephrotic syndrome), bone profile (raised calcium and alkaline phosphatase may indicate bone metastases) and a CEA should all be requested. The latter is not useful in the diagnosis of gastric cancer but may be helpful in detecting recurrence during postoperative follow-up.
- A chest radiograph should be requested to detect metastases.
- A CT scan is used to detect the extent of the tumour and the presence of local and distant metastasis. It may, however, underestimate the extent of regional and distant lymph node metastasis.
- Endoscopic ultrasound has a greater accuracy in early disease in detecting tumour depth and local metastasis compared to an abdominal CT scan.

Staging and prognosis
The TNM staging classification system is used. Only 10–20% of patients have tumours confined to the stomach at presentation. Resection of tumours confined to the mucosa without node metastasis have a 60% 5-year survival, although they account for less than 10% of all tumours. Over half of all tumours have regional and nodal spread at the time of diagnosis (5-year survival less than 15%) and a third have distant metastasis at presentation. The overall 5-year survival for gastric cancer at the time of presentation is 10% in the UK.

Treatment

1. Surgery – curative. Resectable tumours in the distal stomach are best treated with a partial gastrectomy and resection of local lymph nodes. A total gastrectomy is needed for those with larger or more proximal tumours.

2. Surgery – palliative. Palliative surgical procedures are performed for suitable patients with obstruction, intractable pain or bleeding. Palliative total gastrectomy is relatively safe and significantly reduces these symptoms, but has no effect on overall survival. Distal tumours causing obstruction may be bypassed with a gastrojejunostomy, the results of which are unfortunately disappointing. Some proximal tumours causing obstruction can be effectively managed with an endoscopically placed stent or laser ablation procedure.

3. Radiotherapy and chemotherapy. Gastric carcinoma is relatively resistant to radiotherapy; however, moderate doses are sometimes used to palliate complications of local recurrence (e.g. bleeding) or metastasis. For those with locally advanced or metastatic disease, fluorouracil-based chemotherapy regimes have been shown to prolong survival. Furthermore, recent studies have shown that the combination of fluorouracil and radiotherapy after operative resection of locally advanced tumours may prolong survival.

Management of gastric carcinoma in Japan

Japan has the highest incidence of gastric carcinoma in the world; there it is the commonest cause of cancer-related death. The 5-year survival rate for newly diagnosed gastric carcinoma is far higher than in the rest of the world. This could be due to a number of reasons.

- Mass population screening has been implemented with photofluorography followed, if necessary, by endoscopy. Consequently, 40% of newly diagnosed tumours in Japan are potentially curable (compared with 15% in the West).
- Surgical procedures differ in Japan compared to the rest of the world, specifically in the practice of extended radical lymphadenectomy in those with nodal metastasis.
- Operative mortality and morbidity is also significantly lower in the Japanese studies. Part of the reason may be due to the fact that patients are generally younger, thinner and fitter than those in the West. Also, the incidence of proximal and diffuse gastric tumours (which have a poorer prognosis) is higher in the West; and by performing limited nodal resections, the stage of disease may be underestimated, giving a poorer stage-specific survival for western patients.

Primary gastric lymphoma

Gastric lymphoma accounts for less than 5% of all gastric neoplasms, but it is the commonest extranodal lymphoma. The age at presentation is younger than for gastric carcinoma (mean age 36 years old, with a range of 16–68 in a recent review) and the prognosis is generally better.

Clinical features

Clinical features are similar to those of gastric carcinoma but symptoms may be present for months or even years. Weight loss, nausea and vomiting are said to occur earlier than in gastric cancer and haematemesis may be more common. An epigastric mass is present in 30% of cases. Clinical features of nodal lymphoma, such as night sweats and peripheral lymphadenopathy, are typically absent.

Investigations

- Barium meal and endoscopic findings are often indistinguishable from gastric cancer. Polypoid masses on the greater curve, multiple ulcers, thickened rugal folds without luminal narrowing and transpyloric extension into the duodenum are features more in keeping with a lymphoma. Multiple, deep biopsies (using a snare and diathermy) are needed, but diagnostic laparotomy and frozen section biopsies may be necessary to reach a diagnosis.
- Further investigations should include a full blood count, ESR, electrolytes, liver enzymes and chest radiograph.
- Staging investigations include an abdominal CT scan and bone-marrow biopsy (involvement of the bone marrow indicates stage IV disease). Endoscopic ultrasound, if available, is valuable at providing further information.

Staging

The Ann Arbor system of staging is used:

Stage I: Involvement of stomach alone.
Stage II: Localized involvement with its lymph node chain on one side of the diaphragm.
Stage III: Involvement of lymph nodes on both sides of the diaphragm.
Stage IV: Diffuse or disseminated involvement.

Treatment

Treatment regimens have not been standardized, and chemotherapy alone is now more in vogue for early disease. General guidelines are as follows:

1. *Stage I*
- Surgical resection of involved stomach and contiguous structures.
- Radiotherapy has been used for small lesions and for those unsuitable for an operation.
- ?Chemotherapy alone.

2. *Stage II*. Combination radiotherapy and chemotherapy. Surgery is reserved for large, bulky tumours.

3. *Stage III and IV*. Combination chemotherapy with palliative surgery or radiotherapy for obstruction or bleeding.

Eradication of *H. pylori*, if present, may lead to regression in some patients with gastric MALTomas, as may acid-suppression treatment with proton pump inhibitors.

Prognosis   Approximately 50% of patients present in stage I, and the overall 5-year survival rate is 50–60%.

Further reading

Ellis P, Cunningham D. Management of carcinomas of the upper gastrointestinal tract. *British Medical Journal*, 1994; **308**: 834–8.

Fuchs CS, Mayer RJ. Gastric carcinoma. *New England Journal of Medicine*, 1995; **333(1)**: 32–41.

Parsonnet J, Hansen S, Rodriguez L *et al*. *Helicobacter pylori* infection and gastric lymphoma. *New England Journal of Medicine*, 1994; **330**: 1267–71.

Scully RE, Mark EJ, McNeely WF, McNeely BU (eds). Case records of the Massachusetts General Hospital. *New England Journal of Medicine*, 1995; **332**: 1153–9.

Thompson GB, van Heerden JA, Sarr MG. Adenocarcinoma of the stomach: are we making progress? *Lancet*, 1993; **342**: 713–8.

Related topics of interest

MENETRIER'S DISEASE

Menetrier's disease (or hypertrophic gastritis) is a rare disease of unknown aetiology, characterized by giant mucosal folds in the gastric fundus and body. The histological features are of increased mucosal thickness, foveolar hyperplasia, gland atrophy and a mild inflammatory infiltrate.

Clinical features

Men are affected more commonly than women. Presentation is usually after age 50, often with peripheral oedema (owing to protein loss from the stomach), epigastric discomfort, diarrhoea and weight loss.

Investigations

- Blood tests reveal hypoalbuminaemia, and often an iron deficiency anaemia.
- Markedly thickened, nodular rugal folds are found on a barium meal examination. The findings may closely resemble a gastric lymphoma (p. 199).
- An endoscopy confirms the radiological findings and often shows superficial ulceration and erosions. A rapid urease test should be done. In subtle cases the diagnosis may be missed if standard biopsies are taken. It is therefore important to obtain full-thickness biopsies that extend to the submucosa if the diagnosis is suspected.
- Endoscopic ultrasound may help to distinguish between the different causes of giant rugal folds, and is useful in guiding the biopsies, particularly if the disease is localized.
- A CT scan may be needed to exclude other causes (particularly gastric lymphoma) if the diagnosis is not certain.
- A 99m-technecium-labelled serum albumin scan is sometimes used to confirm protein loss from the stomach.

Differential diagnosis

- Giant rugal folds may occur as a normal variant.
- A similar form of the disease occurs in children and is associated with CMV infection (CMV gastropathy).
- Similar clinical and histological changes are seen in the Zollinger–Ellison syndrome and in gastric lymphomas.
- The endoscopic features may be confused with linitus plastica.
- Giant gastric folds are found in the Cronkite–Canada syndrome (with alopecia, nail dystrophy and multiple small-intestinal adenomas).

Treatment

- For those with mild symptoms no specific therapy is needed.
- Most cases regress with acid-suppression therapy (proton pump inhibitors are usually used) and *H. pylori*-eradication therapy in those found to be infected.

- Empirical treatments used with varying success include anticholinergics (e.g. probanthine), octreotide and corticosteroids.
- Some patients progress to atrophic gastritis with an improvement of symptoms.
- A minority of patients eventually require a partial gastrectomy to control hypoalbuminaemia and pain.
- An association with Menetrier's disease and adenocarcinoma is described (possibly partly due to a common link with *H. pylori* infection). The magnitude of this increased risk, and guidelines for follow-up screening, have, however, not been established.

Further reading

Hendrix TR, Yardley JH. Menetrier's disease. *Gut*, 1995; **36(6)**: 945–6.

Related topic of interest

Gastritis and duodenitis (p. 112)

NAUSEA AND VOMITING

The history and examination can often establish the cause of nausea and vomiting. They are commonly a secondary response to another primary disease of the gastrointestinal tract, or to primary CNS disease (including the response of the brainstem vomiting centre to stimuli from drugs, toxins and vestibular disorders). There is therefore usually some other symptom (particulary pain), sign or investigation result pointing to the primary cause; generally speaking, nausea and vomiting without any other associated symptom is rarely organic.

Causes

1. *Gastrointestinal*
   - Peptic ulcer disease.
   - Inflammation (gastritis, duodenitis, pancreatitis, cholangitis/cholecystitis, appendicitis, peritonitis, inflammatory bowel disease).
   - Mechanical obstruction (gastric outlet, small bowel, volvulus, hernia).
   - Motility disorders (diabetic gastroparesis, ileus, non-ulcer dyspepsia, postsurgery, IBS).
   - Infiltrations (lymphoma, amyloidosis).
   - Neoplasms (stomach, small bowel).

2. *Central nervous system*
   - Raised intracranial pressure (e.g. meningitis, cerebrovascular accidents/space-occupying lesions).
   - Bleeding into brainstem cerebrospinal fluid (CSF) space, primary brain stem lesions.
   - Vestibular diseases (Ménière's disease, viral labyrinthitis, motion sickness).
   - Migraine.

3. *Drugs (almost any medication)*
   - Centrally acting (opiates, antiparkinsonian agents).
   - Peripherally acting (NSAIDs, theophylline, antibiotics, antiarrhythmics (particularly digoxin), antiepileptics).
   - Chemotherapy (especially cisplatin, adriamycin, cyclophosphamide).
   - Alcohol.

4. *Metabolic*
   - Uraemia.
   - Acidosis.
   - Diabetes mellitus.
   - Thyroid disorders.
   - Hypercalcaemia.
   - Adrenal insufficiency.
   - Pregnancy.

5. *Infections*
- Gastrointestinal (gastroenteritis, hepatitis).
- Other (meningitis, septicaemia, urinary tract, otitis media).

6. *Malignancy*
- Gastric.
- Ovarian.
- Hypernephroma.
- Paraneoplastic syndrome.

7. *Psychiatric*
- Psychogenic.
- Bulimia, anorexia nervosa.

8. *Other*
- Myocardial infarction.
- Postoperative stomach.
- Intestinal pseudo-obstruction.
- Idiopathic (disordered gastric motility may explain many in this group, but specialized diagnostic tests and expertise are required for diagnosis).

Malignancies, metabolic disorders, motility disorders, and psychiatric problems are groups to particularly consider when nausea and vomiting is chronic, and unexplained by early investigation.

Assessment

1. *History*
- The duration, timing and characteristics (contents and odour) of the vomitus are important.
- A thorough drug and alcohol history is important.

2. *Examination*
- Assess hydration and nutritional status.
- An abdominal examination is required for signs of obstruction, mass or peritonism.
- Conduct a neurological examination for signs of raised intracranial pressure or brainstem signs.

3. *Investigations.* These are guided by the clinical findings.
- Blood tests should be performed for electolytes, renal and liver function, calcium, random glucose, thyroid function and amylase.
- Test for adrenal insufficiency if indicated.
- Erect abdominal X-ray.
- Urinalysis and pregnancy test.
- Endoscopy.
- Motility and gastric emptying studies.

Treatment

1. General measures. If signs of fluid depletion are present (postural hypotension, reduced skin turgor), at least 10% of body fluid has been lost and replacement with i.v. fluids is needed. Evidence of hypochloraemia, hypokalaemia and metabolic alkalosis indicates severe vomiting or pyloric stenosis. The bicarbonate is normal in acute vomiting, but is increased in chronic vomiting due to renal compensation. Early correction of fluids and electrolytes is needed in the elderly and chronically ill.

2. Drug treatment. After fluid losses have been replaced and the cause treated, an antiemetic may be indicated. The specific agent depends on the underlying cause:

- Metoclopramide is a phenothiazine derivative with additional peripheral effects on the gastointestinal tract. It is a dopamine antagonist and acts centrally by blocking the chemoreceptor trigger zone. It acts peripherally by promoting gastric emptying and enhancing LOS tone. It is useful for a wide range of gastro-duodenal, hepatic and biliary diseases including motility disorders, and for emesis induced by opioids, anaesthetics and cytotoxics. The tendency to cause acute dystonic reactions, particularly in young women and the elderly, should not be forgotten.
- Domperidone, like metoclopramide, is a dopaminergic antagonist, but causes less sedation and acute dystonic reactions, as it does not readily cross the blood–brain barrier. Domperidone and metoclopramide are ineffective in treating motion sickness and other vestibular disorders.
- Phenothiazines (e.g. prochlorperazine, haloperidol) are useful in treating nausea associated with metastatic disease, radiation sickness, drug-induced vomiting and vestibular disturbances.
- Antihistamines (e.g cinnarizine, cyclizine, betahistine) are useful for vestibular disturbances, including Ménière's disease. All may cause drowsiness and antimuscarinic side-effects. Promethazine may be used to treat vomiting in pregnancy if other methods have failed.
- Hyoscine is the most effective drug for prevention and treatment of motion sickness but anticholinergic side-effects limit its use.

For cytotoxic drug-induced vomiting the following are useful:

- Intravenous dexamethasone and lorazepam before and after chemotherapy.
- Cyclizine (± haloperidol) in a continuous subcutaneous pump.

- Domperidone suppositories four times daily.
- Ondansetron is a specific 5-HT$_3$-receptor antagonist which can be used orally or intravenously, with or without dexamethasone, for severe emesis. Constipation may limit its long-term use.
- Nabilone is a synthetic cannabinoid which has been shown to be superior to prochlorperazine, but almost all patients experience side-effects (sedation, euphoria, vertigo).

Further reading

Baines MJ. ABC of palliative care. Nausea, vomiting and intestinal obstruction. *British Medical Journal*, 1997; **315**: 1148–50.

Grunberg SM, Hesketh PJ. Control of chemotherapy-induced emesis. *New England Journal of Medicine*, 1993; **329**: 1790–6.

Related topic of interest

Dyspepsia (p. 92)

NEUROENDOCRINE TUMOURS

Gastrointestinal neuroendocrine tumours which give rise to clinical diagnosis in life are all rare, the overall prevalence being approximately 10 in 1 000 000 of population. Neuroendocrine tumours that have been silent in life are far more common (see 'Carcinoid tumours' below). For many subtypes, the pancreas is the most common site of the primary (e.g. insulinoma, gastrinoma, vipoma), with the proximal small bowel accounting for most of the rest. Carcinoid tumours are an exception, with most tumours arising in the appendix/distal small bowel. Neuroendocrine tumours are either sporadic or arise in a familial form, associated with the MEN type 1 syndrome (the latter particularly the case when there are multiple neuroendocrine tumours).

Neuroendocrine tumours usually become clinically apparent due to the effect of the hormones they secrete. Some varieties of neuroendocrine tumours are non-secretory, and these, and the secreting types, *may* produce symptoms due to tumour bulk alone, especially with metastatic spread (usually to the liver). Additionally, the carcinoid type may produce symptoms due to the intense inflammatory reaction that often occurs around even tiny amounts of tumour tissue.

This section covers the more common functioning tumours.

Carcinoid tumours

Carcinoids are neuroendocrine tumours that arise from enterochromaffin cells (so named because of their staining characteristics), usually in the gastrointestinal and respiratory tracts. Although all are potentially malignant, the majority are benign and are common incidental findings at autopsy. Most interest has focused on the minority of carcinoids which are malignant and give rise to the carcinoid syndrome (see below).

Characteristics
- Although they may occur at any site in the gastrointestinal tract, over 95% are found in the small bowel, appendix or rectum. Eighty percent are found within 60 cm of the ileocaecal valve.
- These are usually less than 1 cm in size and are often multiple. The tumours extend away from the lumen to the serosa and regional lymph nodes, which may reach a large size.
- Further spread is to the liver, lung and bone and, more rarely, almost any other organ.

Clinical features
- The majority of appendiceal carcinoids are found at the time of appendicectomy, a minority having contributed to the appendicitis by causing luminal obstruction.
- Carcinoid tumours in the small intestine are rarely symptomatic, but some produce subacute obstruction (in some cases due to intussusception).
- Rectal carcinoids are rare and usually found at the time of proctoscopy.

- Carcinoid tumours may manifest as part of the MEN type 1 syndrome (which includes hyperparathyroidism, anterior pituitary tumours and pancreatic endocrine tumours), and an association exists with neurofibromatosis and pernicious anaemia.

Investigations

- Barium studies of the small bowel may show a smooth swelling or polyp. Multiple ileal polyps are highly suggestive of carcinoids.
- Metastatic mesenteric lymph nodes may calcify and be visualized on an abdominal radiograph.
- An ultrasound scan of the liver may show multiple large deposits of variable echogenicity. An important differential diagnosis is metastatic islet cell carcinoma.
- As carcinoids are typically very vascular, a contrast-enhanced CT scan or hepatic angiogram may provide further useful information.
- Bronchial carcinoids often present as incidental coin lesions on routine chest radiographs, or with signs of bronchial obstruction.

Treatment

- Carcinoid tumours <1 cm in size in the appendix are adequately treated with an appendicectomy. Those greater than 2 cm have a higher risk of metastasis and should be treated with a right hemicolectomy.
- Unlike appendiceal carcinoids, the incidence of metastasis with ileal tumours is high. Such tumours should be excised with a wide margin with resection of local lymph nodes and mesentery.
- Hepatic metastasis can be surgically resected or embolized using radiologically guided techniques.
- Radiotherapy and chemotherapy are generally unsuccessful.

Outcome

The unique feature of small bowel carcinoids is the slow rate of local and distant spread compared to other tumours. Many patients also remain remarkably well despite extensive metastatic disease. Of those with incurable small bowel disease, 50% live for greater than 5 years. Those with liver metastasis have a 30% 5-year survival.

The carcinoid syndrome

This syndrome develops when a carcinoid tumour has metastasized to an area that drains into the systemic circulation: this is almost always the liver. In rare cases, carcinoid tumours outside the gastrointestinal tract produce symptoms without metastasizing. The syndrome usually presents in the sixth decade with signs of metastatic disease (including cachexia and hepatomegaly) and the following clinical features:

1. *Flushing attacks.* This is the most characteristic feature of the carcinoid syndrome and presents as episodic erythema over the upper body. It may be associated with sweating, facial oedema, lacrimation, palpitations and hypertension, and may be provoked by stress or alcohol. Gastric and bronchial carcinoids (foregut carcinoids) produce a more severe flush, which may lead to permanent changes of telangiectasia and morphoea-like thickening of the facial skin.

2. *Diarrhoea.* This is less common than flushing and is said not to occur with gastric carcinoids. Diarrhoea is usually mild, episodic and associated with borborygmi. Subacute small bowel obstruction, due to an ileal carcinoid, should be excluded as a possible underlying cause.

3. *Cardiac manifestations.* A late feature of the carcinoid syndrome (30%), these are produced by progressive fibrosis of the right side of the heart, tricuspid regurgitation and pulmonary stenosis, leading to progressive right heart failure.

4. *Other features.* Fibrosis of the great veins, retroperitoneal fibrosis, asthma and pellagra (photosensitive dermatitis, diarrhoea and neurological signs) are other recognized features.

Pathogenesis

Midgut carcinoids (but not foregut) release large quantities of 5-hydroxytryptamine, while gastric carcinoids release histamines, both of which are responsible for some of the features of the carcinoid syndrome. Other vasoactive peptides, prostaglandins, amines and kinins are also incriminated.

Diagnosis

- The diagnosis should be suspected in anyone presenting with episodic flushing, diarrhoea and hepatomegaly.
- Urinary 5-HIAA levels (24-hour) are used to make the diagnosis. Annual levels are also measured to monitor disease progression. False-positive results may be obtained in those eating foods rich in 5-HT (e.g. bananas, avocados and walnuts) or those taking medication such as methysergide, paracetamol and caffeine. Phenothiazines and tricyclic antidepressants may produce false-negative results.
- Localization of the primary carcinoid tumour may be difficult. A chest radiograph; conventional or spiral CT scan of the chest, abdomen or pelvis; barium studies and endoscopic ultrasound all have a role. In recent years, indium-labelled somatostatin scanning has proved helpful in localizing such tumours.
- The extent of the disease is also assessed with the above tests and an echocardiogram may be useful to detect possible cardiac involvement.

| Treatment | • The carcinoid syndrome is rarely curable; however, effective palliation of symptoms is frequently achievable. |

- The carcinoid syndrome is rarely curable; however, effective palliation of symptoms is frequently achievable.
- Traditionally, cyproheptadine (a 5-HT antagonist) has been used to relieve diarrhoea, and H_1 and H_2 receptor antagonists used for symptomatic relief of gastric carcinoids.
- These and many other agents have largely been superseded by octreotide (a long-acting somatostatin analogue). This is usually well tolerated with few adverse effects, but has to be administered subcutaneously. It may cause discomfort at the injection site and, as it reduces pancreatic secretions, some patients on long-term treatment may require pancreatic supplements. Although many patients develop resistance to the effects of octreotide with time, it alleviates symptoms in 90% and is potentially life saving in the carcinoid crisis, when symptoms become severe and continuous.
- Tumour debulking may be used for those who do not respond to octreotide. This may be achieved by selective hepatic artery embolization, surgical enucleation of large hepatic metastasis or partial hepatectomy. Orthotopic liver transplantation has been performed and results are expected to improve.
- Conventional chemotherapy (streptozotocin and 5-fluorouracil) slows disease progression in 60%. Trials using α-interferon have been encouraging, and it is significantly less toxic.
- Receptor-targeted radiotherapy using radiolabelled octreotide is a new treatment and shows promise.

Prognosis

The mean survival in those with the carcinoid syndrome is about 4–5 years. This is very variable, however, and some patients have survived up to 20 years after diagnosis.

Gastrinoma (Zollinger–Ellison syndrome)

Gastrinomas are gastrin-secreting neuroendocrine tumours of the pancreatic islet cells. Approximately 60% are malignant and about half occur as part of the autosomal dominant MEN type 1 syndrome (pancreatic neuroendocrine tumour, pituitary tumour and hyperparathyroidism). Most occur in the head of the pancreas and duodenal wall, where they are easily overlooked at endoscopy.

Clinical features

- Clinical presentation is at 30–50 years of age and most patients have been symptomatic for less than 2 years.
- Patients present with peptic ulceration, usually in the first part of the duodenum, but often multiple and in unusual sites (distal duodenum, jejunum).

- Complications, including bleeding, perforation and pyloric obstruction, are more frequent than for other causes of peptic ulceration.
- One-third have diarrhoea (due to excess hydrochloric acid) and less common features include steatorrhoea (due to inactivation of pancreatic lipases) and vitamin B_{12} deficiency.

Investigations

- The fasting serum gastrin level is invariably elevated. Other causes of a raised gastrin level include acid-suppression medication (which should be stopped prior to testing), achlorhydria, previous vagotomy, hypercalcaemia and chronic renal failure.
- The secretin test and basal gastric acid measurements are frequently abnormal but are usually not performed routinely.
- Localization is frequently difficult as the tumours are often small and multiple (the latter is usually associated with MEN type 1). Initial localization imaging involves ultrasound and a high-resolution CT scan. Isotope-labelled somatostatin analogue imaging has also recently been found to be useful.
- All patients and their relatives should be screened for associated MEN type 1.

Treatment

Surgical removal is possible in less than 20%; however, high-dose omeprazole (80–120 mg/day) is effective in healing almost all ulcers after a month. Prolonged, symptom-free survival is possible even for those with metastasis.

Those symptomatic with metastatic disease can be treated with streptazocin and 5-fluorouracil. Tumour debulking may be possible with selective hepatic artery embolization or a surgical debulking procedure. Orthotopic liver transplantation is sometimes an option and should be discussed with the appropriate referral centre.

The overall 5-year survival is about 70%.

Insulinoma

This is the most common endocrine tumour of the pancreas with an annual incidence of approximately 1–3 per 1 000 000 of the population. Patients may present at any age, with the majority presenting between the ages of 40 and 45. Of all insulinomas, 20% are multiple, 10% are associated with the MEN type 1 syndrome and 10% are malignant.

Clinical features

- Symptoms are those of spontaneous hypoglycaemia, usually in the morning and late afternoon, and may be worse after alcohol or exercise, and are relieved with eating.

- Neuroglycopenia may present with somnolence, diplopia, confusion, headaches, focal neurological deficit or psychiatric disturbances.
- Adrenergic symptoms secondary to hypoglycaemia include anxiety, palpitations, tremor and sweating.
- The symptoms are often subtle and the diagnosis is usually delayed (or misdiagnosed as a psychiatric illness) for several years.

Diagnosis

- Whipples's triad is still used as the basis of diagnosis:

(1) The symptoms are associated with fasting or exercise.
(2) Hypoglycaemia is present while the symptoms are present.
(3) The symptoms are relieved by glucose.

- The diagnosis is confirmed by admitting the patient and measuring glucose and insulin levels on three mornings after a controlled overnight fast.
- A subnormal glucose and normal insulin suggests the diagnosis. A normal C-peptide excludes exogenous insulin administration, but not sulphonylurea ingestion (the main differential diagnoses being surreptitious administration of insulin or oral hypoglycaemics).
- As the majority of insulinomas are small, accurate localization is often difficult. A dynamic CT scan with contrast is the most sensitive imaging modality. Transabdominal and endoscopic ultrasound scanning are also used.
- Pancreatic angiography and selective pancreatic vein sampling of insulin at different levels will localize the tumour to the head, body or tail of the pancreas. This is often combined with intraoperative ultrasonography to increase accuracy.
- Radiolabelled somatostatin scanning is a recently developed localizing technique which may improve the diagnostic accuracy.
- Calcium levels should be checked episodically to detect associated MEN type 1.

Treatment

- Surgical excision is the only effective cure for non-metastasized tumours.
- For metastasized tumours (5–10%), tumours unable to be localized, and for patients with a poor operative risk and mild symptoms, medical therapy is used. This entails a combination of dietary advice (eating regular high-carbohydrate meals), and medication (principally diazoxide or octreotide).

Glucagonoma

Glucagonomas usually occur between the ages of 50 and 70. Most have metastasized to the liver by the time of diagnosis.

Clinical features The characteristic syndrome consists of:

- Necrolytic migratory erythema, which is a superficial bullous eruption which begins in the intertrigenous areas and waxes and wanes, involving various different anatomical sites. The rash often precedes the diagnosis by several years.
- Glucose intolerance (or overt diabetes) is common and usually precedes the diagnosis by many years.
- Weight loss. This may be profound and occurs with small non-metastasized tumours.
- Other features include a normochromic normocytic anaemia and an increased incidence of thromboembolic episodes, diarrhoea and depression.

Diagnosis
- Hyperglucagonaemia with suggestive clinical features is diagnostic. A raised plasma glucagon level is also found in various other conditions (e.g. chronic renal failure, prolonged starvation, acute pancreatitis, diabetic ketoacidosis) but the levels are seldom as high as with a glucagonoma.
- Most tumours are large at the time of diagnosis (5–10 cm) and are best localized with a CT scan.

Treatment
- Surgery should be considered in all patients regardless of tumour stage. Although resection of localized tumours is potentially curative, most have spread at the time of diagnosis. Surgical tumour debulking may palliate symptoms in such cases.
- Subcutaneous octreotide alleviates the rash, diarrhoea and weight loss in the majority of patients, although the beneficial effects may wane with time. Streptozotocin is a further option for metastatic disease.

Vipoma (Verner–Morrison syndrome)

- The characteristic syndrome occurs as a result of the excessive secretion of VIP by a neuroendocrine tumour of the pancreas.
- Most occur in middle age or the elderly and are large (>3 cm) and in the tail of the pancreas.
- Two-thirds of vipomas are malignant.
- The cardinal features of the syndrome are:
  Watery diarrhoea, which is often profuse, but may be intermittent in the early stages.

Hypokalaemia.

Achlorhydria (usually with a metabolic acidosis).

Weight loss is almost invariably present and facial flushing occurs in some patients.

Diagnosis
- The diagnosis is made with the finding of an elevated fasting plasma VIP concentration in the presence of a secretory diarrhoea (usually >3 l/day).
- Ultrasonography (percutaneous or endoscopic), contrast-enhanced CT scanning or angiography will detect most vipomas.

Treatment
- Correction of fluid and electrolyte losses is the first line in management.
- Octreotide ameliorates the diarrhoea in the majority of patients.
- Surgical resection is warranted in those without metastatic disease. Surgical debulking procedures have not been evaluated.

Further reading

Basson MD, Ahlman H, Wangberg B, Modlin IM. Biology and management of the midgut carcinoid. *American Journal of Surgery*, 1993; **165(2)**: 288–97.

Modlin IM, Lewis JJ, Ahlman H *et al*. Management of unresectable malignant endocrine tumours of the pancreas. *Surgery, Gynecology and Obstetrics*, 1993; **176(5)**: 507–18.

Norton JA. Neuroendocrine tumours of the pancreas and duodenum. *Current Problems in Surgery*, 1994; **31(2)**: 77–156.

Related topic of interest

Diarrhoea (p. 81)

OESOPHAGEAL CARCINOMA

Oesophageal carcinoma is one of the most lethal carcinomas. It has a median survival of 10 months at diagnosis, and a cure rate of less than 5%; much better outcomes have been reported in Japanese studies. Worldwide, the majority are squamous carcinomas, which are about four times more common than adenocarcinomas. Within, and between, countries the incidence of squamous carcinoma varies dramatically, suggesting strong environmental factors in causation. Adenocarcinoma of the oesophagus is largely a disease of developed countries; the incidence of it has risen rapidly over the last 20 years (faster than for any other tumour). Adenocarcinomas tend to spread to the lymph nodes early and are more poorly differentiated at presentation than squamous carcinomas.

Causes

- The cause of squamous cell carcinoma is unknown, but a strong link is found with the ingestion of certain substances, including tobacco, alcohol, nitrosamines and aflatoxin-contaminated cereals. Human papillomavirus and *Aspergillus* are possible associated infectious agents. Diets deficient in vitamins A, C and E, riboflavin or trace metals (zinc, molybdenum and magnesium) are also associated with an increased risk.
- Medical conditions associated with an increased risk of squamous cell carcinomas include corrosive injury, achalasia, Plummer–Vinson syndrome (postcricoid web and iron deficiency anaemia), familial tylosis (type A), systemic sclerosis and CD.
- Incidence rates vary widely around the world and in different ethnic groups. The highest incidence is found in northern China, parts of Iran (the 'Asian oesophageal cancer belt') and Transkei (South Africa). Although it is one of the most common cancers worldwide, it accounts for only 2% of cancer deaths in the UK annually.
- Adenocarcinomas usually arise from areas of classic Barrett's oesophagus or from short segments of columnar metaplasia in the distal oesophagus – metaplastic changes which, in turn, have arisen as a consequence of GORD. Why some patients with a columnar-lined oesophagus develop adenocarcinoma and others do not is poorly understood.

Clinical features

- Patients usually present in the seventh to eighth decades with the recent onset of progressive dysphagia. This indicates that approximately two-thirds of the circumference of the wall is involved and that the disease is likely to be incurable. Dysphagia developing in a patient in this age group should always be considered to be due to an oesophageal cancer until proven otherwise.

	• Other symptoms include weight loss, retrosternal discomfort, odynophagia, sialorrhoea, chest infections (from regurgitation or oesophagopulmonary fistula), bleeding, hoarseness (sometimes due to recurrent laryngeal nerve involvement) or hiccups (suggesting diaphragmatic spread).
Investigations	• Diagnosis initially involves a double-contrast barium swallow, which will show the extent of the lesion and may detect occult tumours in the hypopharynx or cardia. • Endoscopic assessment enables a biopsy and/or brush cytology to be performed. It also allows endoscopic dilatation (see below) to relieve dysphagia, whilst awaiting the results of confirmatory and staging investigations. • Blood tests should include a full blood count (to detect anaemia from occult bleeding), electrolytes (may show signs of dehydration), liver enzymes (indicating possible metastases) and serum calcium.
Staging investigations	The TNM system of staging is used. Relevant staging investigations include a chest radiograph (which may show a widened superior mediastinum from local spread or, rarely, lung metastases), a CT scan of the chest (to detect local lymph node spread) and abdomen (to detect the presence of liver metastases), and a lymph node biopsy (to confirm metastases). In cases with minimal extraluminal spread as detected by a CT scan, endoscopic ultrasonography is the single most reliable staging procedure to determine operability. If endoscopic ultrasonography is unavailable, a laparoscopy may be indicated.
Treatment	• Unfortunately, less than 10% of patients present with potentially curable disease (i.e. confined to the mucosa or submucosa). In this group, certain centres are able to achieve a 60–80% 5-year survival with radical surgical procedures. • For locally advanced adenocarcinoma, recent evidence has shown a significant survival benefit of preoperative chemotherapy (fluorouracil and cisplatin) with radiotherapy over surgery alone. Preoperative radiotherapy without chemotherapy has not been shown to be of benefit.
	Patients with irresectable tumours have a mean survival of about 4–6 months. Death is usually due to local complications (e.g. aspiration pneumonia) rather than to effects of distant metastases.
	Palliation of malignant dysphagia. There is no single, ideal palliative procedure, and management should be tailored to the individual, and to local facilities/expertise. Some patients

require a combination of therapies, depending on the natural history of the disease process. Temporary relief of dysphagia can be achieved a number of ways:

- Peroral dilatation can be achieved with a number of different rigid dilators or hydrostatic through-the-scope dilators. These procedures can be repeated when dysphagia returns.
- Endoscopic thermal (YAG) laser photodestruction can be performed as an out-patient procedure. It is effective (over 80% of patients are able to swallow normal food after the procedure), safe (it has a 1% mortality rate and a 4% complication rate) and may prolong the mean survival. The main disadvantage over stent insertion is the need for repetitive treatments and the cost of recurrent day-case admissions. To reduce the number of interventions, laser treatment has been combined with radiotherapy or photodynamic therapy (see below).
- Alcohol injections into exophytic tumours is cheap and easy to perform, but not as effective as other local destructive procedures.
- A semi-rigid oesophageal endoprosthesis (Celestin or Atkinson tube) is often used for distal malignant oesophageal strictures. Insertion is associated with a mortality rate of up to 13%, and a morbidity of 15%. Complications include tumour overgrowth, tube migration, reflux with or without aspiration, and perforation. Swallowing is never normal, and patients are only able to tolerate pureed foods.
- Self-expanding metal stents are becoming increasingly popular for both distal and more proximal lesions. They are associated with fewer complications than rigid intubation, and the procedure-related mortality is about 2%. Metallic stents are, however, 10 times as expensive as conventional rigid tubes, and five times as expensive as laser therapy. Tumour overgrowth at the ends of the stent, or ingrowth between the mesh of the stent, causes re-stenosis in 5–20% of patients. This rate of recurrent dysphagia is about the same as for rigid stents. The development of coated metal stents may have overcome some of these problems.
- Some series have shown excellent short-term palliation of symptoms with external beam radiotherapy, or internal radiotherapy (brachytherapy), with or without chemotherapy.
- Radical radiotherapy alone is used for proximal squamous cell tumours but relieves dysphagia in less than half (and has a high incidence of side-effects).

- Laser photocoagulation therapy or thermal ablation with bipolar probes are used in some centres.
- A percutaneous enterogastric feeding tube is an option for those who are unable to maintain an adequate nutritional intake.

Further reading

Chung SCS, Stuart RC, Li AKC. Surgical therapy for squamous-cell carcinoma of the oesophagus. *Lancet*, 1994; **343**: 521–4.

Ellis P, Cunningham D. Management of carcinomas of the upper gastrointestinal tract. *British Medical Journal*, 1994; **308**: 834–8.

Hennessy TPJ. Cancer of the oesophagus. *Postgraduate Medical Journal*, 1996; **72**: 458–63.

Sturgess RP, Morris AI. Metal stents in the oesophagus. *Gut*, 1995; **37**: 593–4.

Walsh NW, Noonan N, Hollywood D, Kelly A, Stat C, Keeling N. A comparison of multimodal therapy and surgery for oesophageal adenocarcinoma. *New England Journal of Medicine*, 1996; **335(7)**: 462–7.

Related topics of interest

Barrett's oesophagus (p. 22)
Dysphagia (p. 98)

OESOPHAGEAL DYSMOTILITY

Oesophageal motility disorders may be either primary or secondary.

Primary disorders include achalasia and diffuse oesophageal spasm. *Secondary* causes are numerous and include connective tissue diseases (particularly systemic sclerosis), neurological diseases (cerebrovascular accident, motor neurone disease, multiple sclerosis), primary muscular diseases (myasthenia gravis, myotonic dystrophy) and neuropathies (diabetes, alcohol).

Diffuse oesophageal spasm

This condition is caused by intermittent, irregular non-peristaltic contractions of the oesophagus in the absence of any organic cause. It occurs in both sexes at any age, but is most common over the age of 50.

Clinical features

Patients complain of two symptoms: dysphagia and chest pain.

- Dysphagia is intermittent, occurs with both liquids and solids, is variable in severity and is usually accompanied by pain.
- Chest pain is usually precipitated by a meal or emotional stress. It may be mild or severe and may mimic cardiac pain (and like cardiac pain, may be relieved by nitrates). The term 'nutcracker oesophagus' is used to describe a condition in which rapid high-amplitude peristaltic contractions in the oesophagus produce angina-like chest pain with or without dysphagia.

Investigations

- A barium swallow may reveal changes of segmental non-peristaltic contractions producing what is described as a 'corkscrew' or 'rosary bead' oesophagus. Another less common finding is a tight contraction of the mid-oesophagus with a slight dilatation proximally, but unlike achalasia, no stasis of food is found. As the symptoms are episodic, the barium swallow is often normal and any abnormality present bears no correlation to the severity of symptoms (similar features are found in the asymptomatic elderly).
- An endoscopy is needed to exclude other causes of dysphagia.
- Those with persistent symptoms and a normal barium swallow should be referred for oesophageal manometry. Manometric studies show repetitive wave forms (several peaks after a single swallow) in most patients and spontaneous contractions (peaks not induced by swallowing) in over half. The test is useful if positive, but a negative test does not exclude the diagnosis. Sensitivity of the test may be improved with ambulatory studies or provocation stimuli (using edrophonium or infused acid) to trigger oesophageal contraction.

Treatment	Treatment is often unrewarding. Reassurance of the benign nature of the disease is important to allay anxiety. Long-acting oral nitrates (or a sternal nitrate patch) may be effective, but side-effects and tolerance limit their long-term use. Calcium channel blockers (particularly nifedipine) have been shown to decrease the severity of contractions but their clinical efficacy is controversial.

For occasional cases where dysphagia is a prominent feature, and manometry has confirmed high-amplitude contractions, pneumatic dilatation can be tried. The outcome is unpredictable and the risk of perforation with the procedure should be borne in mind.

Irritable oesophagus

- This condition is believed to be due to lower oesophageal hypersensitivity to normal stimuli (e.g. refluxed gastric acid), or possibly to an underlying motility disorder.
- It presents as atypical retrosternal chest pain (which may closely mimic angina). The pain, unlike stable angina, often occurs at rest and is associated with dysphagia. It is a relatively common cause of dysphagia in the elderly.
- Endoscopy is normal, but is important to rule out other causes of dysphagia.
- The diagnosis is sometimes confirmed with a 24-hour ambulatory oesophageal pH, which may show that symptoms coincide with periods of oesophageal acid exposure, even though, overall, this exposure may lie within the normal range (i.e. a cumulative period when distal oesophageal pH falls below 4 that is less than 5% of the total, 24-hour recording period).
- Less reliable (and largely obsolete) provocation tests include Bernstein's acid infusion test (for reflux) and the balloon distension test and edrophonium test (for motility disorders).
- Treatment is not often successful. Depending on the underlying abnormality, either acid suppression or smooth muscle relaxants (such as nitrates or calcium channel blockers) should be tried. Drugs that alter pain perception (such as tricyclic antidepressants) are occasionally beneficial, but they should be used with caution in the elderly.

Further reading

British Society of Gastroenterology Guidelines in Gastroenterology. Guidelines for oesophageal manometry and pH monitoring, September 1996.

Vantrappen GR, Janssens J. Motility disorders. In: Bouchier IAD, Allen RN, Hodgson HJF, Keighley MRB (eds). *Gastroenterology – Clinical Science and Practice*, 2nd edn. Philadelphia: WB Saunders, 1993; 69–81.

Vantrappen G, Janssens J, Ghillebert G. The irritable oesophagus – a frequent cause of angina-like pain. *Lancet*, 1987; **1**: 1232–4.

Related topic of interest

Dysphagia (p. 98)

OESOPHAGEAL WEBS, RINGS AND DIVERTICULA

Oesophageal webs

- An 'oesophageal web' is a thin 2–3 mm mucosal structure, extending from part of the wall of the oesophagus into the lumen. Unlike oesophageal rings, they are not circumferential.
- They may be either congenital or acquired. Congenital webs usually occur in the mid- or lower oesophagus. They may present as dysphagia, or more commonly are found incidentally at endoscopy or barium swallow.
- Idiopathic or acquired webs are usually postcricoid. Acquired webs may be due to chronic graft-versus-host disease, epidermolysis bullosa, or as part of the Patterson–Brown–Kelly syndrome. The latter occurs almost exclusively in middle-aged women, and presents as an iron deficiency anaemia, postcricoid web (producing high dysphagia), and predisposes to high oesophageal carcinoma.
- An endoscopy and barium swallow may miss small webs, particularly those in the upper oesophagus, in which case cineradiology is the preferred investigation.
- An ear, nose and throat (ENT) opinion may be necessary to assess those with high dysphagia.
- Treatment is with endoscopic balloon dilatation.

Oesophageal rings

- Oesophageal rings are thicker circumferential structures involving mucosa and muscle. They usually occur in the lower oesophagus.
- Schatzki's ring, a submucosal band at the squamocolumnar junction, is the most common. The aetiology is uncertain, but some may be related to GORD. They are usually detected incidentally on a barium swallow, or less often by endoscopy. Symptomatic patients usually complain of intermittent dysphagia, signifying that the lumen is less than 20 mm in diameter. Such patients may experience intermittent complete oesophageal obstruction after eating bread or meat (the 'steakhouse syndrome'). Symptomatic patients should be investigated with a barium meal.
- Endoscopic biopsy is indicated, and those patients with dysphagia are best treated with endoscopic balloon dilatation.
- For those patients with large webs which are unable to be dilated, electrosurgical incision with sphincterotome or YAG laser has been successfully used.
- Acid-suppression therapy has been used after dilatation, but the benefit is unproven.

Oesophageal diverticula

Oesophageal diverticula occur in one of three areas:

- Immediately above the upper oesophageal sphincter in the pharynx – pharyngeal pouch (Zenker's diverticulum).

- In the mid-oesophagus – either pulsion or traction diverticula.
- Immediately above the LOS – epiphrenic diverticula.

Zenker's diverticulum
- This is the commonest form of diverticulum.
- It arises from a dehiscence between the cricopharyngeus and inferior constrictor muscles.
- Patients are usually elderly, and complain of transient high dysphagia with aspiration or regurgitation of food.
- The diagnosis is confirmed by a barium swallow. Endoscopy should be avoided due to the risk of perforation.
- Those with troublesome symptoms are treated surgically. The operation of choice is a cricopharyngeal myotomy with diverticulopexy or excision of the diverticulum.

Mid-oesophageal diverticula
- These are usually incidental findings.
- Any symptoms are usually due to underlying oesophageal dysmotility or GORD.
- Treatment of underlying GOR or dysmotility is appropriate and surgery is rarely necessary.

Epiphrenic diverticula
- These may be found incidentally at endoscopy or barium meal, or in association with motor abnormalities of the lower oesophagus (usually achalasia).
- Nocturnal regurgitation of fluid is characteristic, but whether it is from the diverticulum or underlying achalasia is debatable.
- The diagnosis may be missed at endoscopy, and is confirmed with a barium swallow.
- The treatment is of the underlying condition, with surgical diverticular excision if it is large.

Further reading

Pope CE II. Rings, webs, diverticula. In: Sleisenger MH, Fordtran JS (eds). *Gastrointestinal Disease – Pathophysiology/Diagnosis/Management*, 5th edn. Philadelphia: WB Saunders, 1993; 419–27.

Related topic of interest

Dysphagia (p. 98)

PORTAL HYPERTENSION

Portal hypertension arises due to an increased resistance to portal vein blood flow, which may occur anywhere along the course of the portal vein.

The causes are classified into three main groups.

Prehepatic
- Increased splenic blood flow (e.g. arteriovenous fistulae).
- Portal vein thrombosis (due to e.g. umbilical infection in neonates, appendicitis or peritonitis in older children, inflammatory bowel disease, biliary tract infections, hypercoagulable states, posthepatobiliary surgery, trauma, invasion by tumour (e.g. hepatocellular or pancreatic carcinoma), retroperitoneal fibrosis). Fifty percent of cases are idiopathic.
- Splenic vein thrombosis (e.g. postsplenectomy, chronic pancreatitis, carcinoma of the pancreas).

Intrahepatic
1. *Presinusoidal*
- Schistosomiasis (the commonest cause worldwide).
- Sarcoidosis.
- Myeloproliferative disease.
- Chronic active hepatitis.
- Toxins (e.g. polyvinyl chloride, copper, arsenic).
- Congenital hepatic fibrosis.

2. *Sinusoidal*
- Cirrhosis (the commonest cause in the West).
- Non cirrhotic causes (e.g. acute alcoholic hepatitis, cytotoxic drugs, vitamin A intoxication).

Posthepatic
- Veno-occlusive disease.
- Budd–Chiari syndrome.
- Increased right atrial pressure (e.g. constrictive pericarditis).

Consequences of portal hypertension
- With intrahepatic portal obstruction, collateral vessels form between portal vessels and systemic circulation veins. These are found in four main sites:
  - Group I: (a) at the fundus of the stomach and lower oesophagus, and (b) ano-rectum.
  - Group II: In the falciform ligament of the liver.
  - Group III: In the retroperitoneal tissue or anterior abdominal wall (including scars of previous operations).
  - Group IV: At the left renal vein.
- With extrahepatic portal venous obstruction, collaterals form in an attempt to bypass the block and return blood to the liver. They are most prominent at the hepatic hilum, in

the suspensory ligament of the liver, in the diaphragm and at the omentum.

- The most important consequence of portal hypertension is the development of, and subsequent bleeding from, gastro-oesophageal varices. Other consequences are ascites (p. 14), splenomegaly and hypersplenism, and portal hypertensive gastropathy.

Clinical features

- Haematemesis from bleeding oesophageal varices is the commonest presentation. This may precipitate hepatic encephalopathy in those with hepatic causes, but not with prehepatic causes, as hepatocellular function is usually preserved in this group. Haematemesis is occasionally secondary to portal hypertensive gastropathy, which is exacerbated following repeated episodes of oesophageal variceal sclerotherapy. Stigmata of chronic liver disease will be evident in hepatic causes.
- Collateral veins radiating outwards from the umbilicus (caput Medusae) are rare, and only seen if the umbilical vein remains patent. They are distinguished from dilated abdominal wall collaterals seen in inferior vena cava obstruction as, with the latter, flow in the veins below the umbilicus is upwards.
- A venous hum or thrill may be detected beneath the xiphisternum or at the umbilicus (due to collaterals in the falciform ligament).
- Splenomegaly is invariable, and pancytopenia (indicative of hypersplenism) may be present in long-standing cases.
- A small, firm liver is suggestive of cirrhosis; an enlarged soft liver is more typical of extrahepatic portal venous obstruction.

Investigations

- Chronic liver disease should be confirmed with a liver biopsy, and the cause established with the necessary investigations (p. 41).
- Endoscopy is the best method of visualizing oesophageal and gastric varices. They may be graded as follows:

    Grade I varices are barely visible.
    Grade II varices protrude into less than 10% of the lumen.
    Grade III varices protrude into 50% or more of the lumen.
    Large varices and those with cherry-red spots are most likely to bleed.

- Ultrasound usually shows a dilated portal vein and collaterals in portal hypertension. Portal vein thrombosis can also be ascertained.
- Doppler ultrasound is useful in showing the anatomy of, and flow in, the portal veins and hepatic artery. Colour

Doppler is accurate in showing portosystemic shunts and in the diagnosis of the Budd–Chiari syndrome.

- If portal surgery or liver transplantation is being considered, or if the ultrasound shows a probable thrombosed portal vein, more accurate information is obtained with venography. The coeliac axis is catheterized via the femoral artery and the splenic artery and superior mesenteric artery are injected with contrast. The portal vein pressure is determined by measuring the wedged hepatic venous pressure, by inserting a balloon catheter into a hepatic vein radicle via the femoral vein. The normal portal pressure is 5–6 mmHg, and in alcoholic cirrhosis, levels above 12 mmHg are associated with an increased risk of bleeding from oesophgeal varices (see below).

Management

Treatment is aimed at the underlying cause (e.g. alcohol abstinence in alcoholic cirrhosis, anticoagulants for thrombophilia, steroids for autoimmune hepatitis, etc.) and the complications (principally bleeding oesophageal varices and ascites).

1. Oesophageal varices – prevention of bleeding

- The likelihood of the varices bleeding is dependent on the size of varices (the larger the varix, the more likely it is to bleed), the presence and number of red spots on the varices, the portal pressure (increased risk if >12 mmHg) and the Child's grade of hepatocellular function (see p. 42).
- Propranolol, in a dose which reduces the resting pulse by 25%, lowers the portal pressure in up to two-thirds of patients, and reduces the risk of bleeding (but has no effect on mortality). The response is, however, very variable, particularly in those with advanced cirrhosis. Wedge hepatic venous pressure measurements allow objective measurement of the response and thus the likelihood of benefit, but are available only in specialist centres.
- Isosorbide-mononitrate is as effective as propranolol and may be used in those in whom β-blockers are contraindicated. Used together, they have an additive effect.
- In general, endoscopic sclerotherapy is not beneficial for the primary prophylaxis of bleeding due to an unacceptable complication rate. Endoscopic band ligation (see below) does, however, show promise as a primary prophylaxis, particularly for large varices.
- After an episode of bleeding, re-bleeding rates can be reduced by a course of endoscopic therapy (either injection sclerotherapy or band ligation) to obliterate the varices. Although this reduces the number of re-bleeds, the overall mortality is unaltered. Treatments are usualy repeated at 2-weekly intervals until the varices are obliterated. The

optimum frequency and duration of subsequent follow-up endoscopy is not certain, and depends in part on local resources: 30–40% of varices return each year after therapy is stopped.

2. *Management of bleeding varices*

- Patients may present with melaena and anaemia indicating a slow bleed, or with a sudden haematemesis. Both forms of bleeding may worsen an underlying hepatic encephalopathy.
- Resuscitation with i.v. colloid, blood or dextrose (saline should be avoided) is the first priority. Over-resuscitation should be avoided as over-expansion of the blood volume may precipitate further bleeding.
- A coagulation abnormality should be corrected with fresh frozen plasma and a single i.v. dose of 10 mg of vitamin K (repeat doses have no additional benefit).
- Endoscopy should be performed urgently to confirm the source of bleeding and to perform sclerotherapy. It is important to remember that up to one-third of patients with known varices bleed from other sites, usually DU, gastric erosions and Mallory–Weiss tears.
- Endoscopic injection sclerotherapy is performed by injecting up to 4 ml of 5% ethanolamine (or other sclerosant) into each varix. This is effective at controlling the acute bleed in up to 90% of cases. Re-bleeding occurs in about 30% of patients and further sclerotherapy is warranted. If bleeding recurs following a second course of sclerotherapy, other measures should be used (see below). Many patients experience some chest pain, fever and dysphagia after sclerotherapy. Other complications include mediastinitis, bleeding from the injection site, perforation and stricture formation. Clinical presentation of perforation may occur 5–7 days after injection sclerotherapy, seen as mediastinal air on a chest radiograph, or a pneumothorax. Complications can be reduced by avoiding the use of excessive volumes of sclerosant.
- Endoscopic variceal band ligation is as effective as injection, and causes less complications. However, it is technically more difficult to perform in the presence of active bleeding. It should be the treatment of choice once active bleeding has been controlled, and for secondary prophylaxis.
- Medical therapy to lower portal pressure is used in all patients as an adjunct to sclerotherapy. It can be instituted immediately when variceal bleeding is suspected, and requires no special expertise or equipment. Intravenous

octreotide (a long-acting somatostatin analogue), at a dose of 50 μg stat, then 50 μg/hour over 72 hours, is the treatment of choice. Vasopressin or terlipressin (which cause splanchnic arteriolar vasoconstriction) plus i.v./transdermal nitroglycerin (to prevent vasopressin-induced coronary vasoconstriction and to further reduce variceal pressure) is an alternative, and may be more effective.

- If bleeding persists after medical therapy plus injection sclerotherapy, oesophageal tamponade with a Sengstaken–Blakemore tube (or equivalent) will rapidly achieve control in 90% of cases. The tube consists of two balloons: the distal one is inflated in the stomach with at least 250 ml of air and pulled up to abut the gastro-oesophageal junction; the proximal balloon can be inflated in the oesophagus, with the pressure between 50–60 mmHg as measured by a sphygmomanometer. The oesophageal balloon should only be used if adequate haemostasis is not obtained with the gastric balloon, as it carries a risk of oesophageal ulceration and pressure necrosis, particularly if inflated for >8 hours. There is a lumen for aspiration in the oesophagus above the balloon which should be continuous, and one for gastric aspiration, which should be hourly. Complications include upper airway obstruction, aspiration pneumonia (prevented by tube aspiration, as above) and perforation. The Linton tube is safer, but perhaps less well known. There is a single gastric balloon inflated with up to 600 ml of air, and kept under tension with a 1 kg weight (e.g. a litre bag of i.v. fluid).

- For those patients that continue to bleed, a percutaneously inserted TIPSS can be used. These have largely replaced surgical shunts, as they are easier to insert and are associated with fewer complications, and do not preclude subsequent hepatic transplantation (they are often used as a temporizing measure whilst awaiting a transplant). The main complications are stent occlusion (affecting over 60% at 2 years) and hepatic encephalopathy (which occurs in 25–30%).

- If bleeding cannot be controlled with a Sengstaken–Blakemore tube and/or TIPSS placement, emergency surgery is needed. These procedures carry a high mortality rate, particularly in patients with end-stage liver disease. Oesophageal transection, using a staple gun under general anaesthesia, is usually used. This almost invariably stops further haemorrhage. An emergency surgical portosystemic shunt may be created between a portal vessel and the inferior vena cava using either a side-to-side anastomosis or a dacron graft. In cases of end-stage liver disease and uncontrollable variceal haemorrhage, liver transplantation can be considered.

- In addition to the control of bleeding, lactulose should be used to empty the bowels of blood (in oral and enema form in doses that produce frequent loose stools) as, although unpleasant for all concerned, this reduces the risk of hepatic encephalopathy. Intravenous antibiotics are also administered, as such patients have a high risk of sepsis (usually from aspiration pneumonia or peritonitis).

Further reading

Stanley AJ, Hayes PC. Portal hypertension and variceal haemorrhage. *Lancet*, 1997; **350**: 1235–9.
Williams SG, Westaby D. Management of variceal haemorrhage. *British Medical Journal*, 1994; **308**: 1213–17.

Related topics of interest

Ascites (p. 14)
Cirrhosis (p. 40)
Haematemesis and melaena (p. 135)

POSTSURGICAL STOMACH

The number of upper gastrointestinal operations for peptic ulcer disease has declined sharply since the introduction of H_2 receptor antagonists in the 1970s. Anatomical and physiological derangements are common in the first few weeks after surgery, and depend on the extent of surgery. Division of the vagus nerve and ablation or bypass of the pylorus are the most important factors contributing to postgastrectomy syndromes. Overall, 20% of patients are left with long-term symptoms.

It is useful to consider the stomach as having two distinct physiological motor areas.

- The proximal stomach is involved with regulating intragastric pressure and gastric emptying of liquids. Operations that impair proximal gastric function may cause rapid gastric emptying of liquids and, subsequently, dumping and diarrhoea.
- The distal stomach, with its peristaltic contractions, has a major role in the mixing and emptying of solids. Operations affecting distal gastric contractions, such as truncal vagotomy, may impede gastric emptying of solids and cause gastric atony.

Specific postsurgical problems are listed below.

Diarrhoea

- This most commonly complicates truncal vagotomy, although it may occur after any gastric surgery. It is thought to be due to a faster gastric emptying time and the rapid entry of hypertonic liquid into the small bowel, which overloads its absorptive capacity. A more rapid small bowel transit time is also thought to be a factor.
- Typically patients complain of diarrhoea within 1 or 2 hours of eating.
- Other causes of diarrhoea should be excluded (e.g. CD, immunoglobulin deficiency and small bowel bacterial overgrowth).
- Treatment involves eating smaller, more frequent meals and medical treatment with loperamide, codeine phosphate or cholestyramine.

Gastric stasis

- This manifests as postprandial bloating, early satiety and vomiting of partially digested food. It may be due to disordered motility (particularly after vagotomy), mechanical obstruction of the afferent loop or a stomal ulcer.
- A barium meal and endoscopy are helpful in reaching a diagnosis. Coexisting conditions which produce similar symptoms (e.g. cholelithiasis) should also be considered.
- Medical treatment with prokinetic agents (e.g. domperidone or cisapride) and advising a more liquid diet may be useful in cases of altered motility.
- Mechanical obstruction is treated surgically.

Bile (or alkaline) reflux gastritis

- This occurs when duodenal contents reflux into the stomach causing gastritis and sometimes bilious vomiting, particularly in the morning. It may occur immediately after surgery or years later. It is particularly a feature after the Billroth II operation.

- Endoscopy may reveal gastritis, but the presence of duodeno-gastric reflux is difficult to confirm. An isotope scan of biliary excretion ('HIDA' scan) can provide useful information.
- Prokinetic agents, sucralfate, cholestyramine and aluminium-containing antacids can all be tried.
- Surgical revision is indicated for severe cases.

Dumping

This may be divided into two types: early and late.

Early dumping

- Early dumping is characterized by epigastric fullness, sweating, faintness and palpitations 30 min after eating. It results from rapid gastric emptying which produces a hypertonic load in the small bowel, thus triggering autonomic reflexes and the release of vasoactive peptides (VIP and neurotensin in particular).
- Relief may be obtained by eating smaller meals that are low in sugar and high in fibre. Prescribing fluids between, rather than with, meals may also help.
- The addition of colloids, such as guar or pectin, to the diet may help by reducing the rate of delivery of carbohydrate to the small intestine. Subcutaneous octreotide (a somatostatin analogue) may be useful in the short term by reducing neuroendocrine secretions and gastrointestinal motility. Tolerance is a problem with long-term use.

Late dumping

- This occurs 2–3 hours after a meal and is caused by rebound hypoglycaemia after rapid carbohydrate absorption has stimulated excessive or asynchronous insulin secretion.
- Treatment options are the same as for early dumping. Surgical revision is considered only for the most resistant cases.

Recurrent dyspepsia

After an operation for peptic ulcer disease, the symptoms may recur. An endoscopy is indicated to detect the recurrence of the ulcer or development of a carcinoma. If an ulcer is present, it should be biopsied and the Zollinger–Ellison syndrome excluded with plasma gastrin levels (remembering that a vagotomy and antisecretory agents all cause hypergastrinaemia). Treatment with a proton pump inhibitor is effective for those ulcers not caused by duodeno-gastric reflux. The completeness of a vagotomy may be checked by cephalic-stimulated acid-secretion studies, although this may be difficult to interpret in the presence of duodeno-gastric reflux.

If no ulcer is present, cholelithiasis should be excluded and treatment for non-ulcer dyspepsia given.

Weight loss

Weight loss is a relatively common problem after gastric surgery and usually is accounted for by a reduced dietary intake. Less common causes include chronic gastric outlet obstruction (due to pyloric stenosis or bezoars), gastric stasis or malabsorption (discussed below).

Malabsorption

- For patients with weight loss and loose stools after gastric surgery, the following favour malabsorption over simple postgastrectomy dysfunction:
    Increased fecal fat excretion (<9 g/day is normal and >15 g/day is significant).
    Hypoproteinaemia.
    Prolonged INR.
    Reduced vitamin B_{12} level.
- Causes include bacterial overgrowth in the proximal small bowel (blind loop syndrome), pancreatic atrophy (this occurs in some patients many years after gastric resections for reasons that are unclear; the simplest confirmatory test is a therapeutic response to pancreatic enzyme supplements), rapid intestinal emptying due to global dysmotility, and recurrence of disease.
- The diagnosis of bacterial overgrowth is made by a quantitative culture of small bowel contents; however, a therapeutic trial of antibiotics is usually a more practical approach.
- Endoscopy, barium meal follow-through study and possibly colonoscopy are used to detect recurrence of Crohn's disease.
- Surgical revision may be required.

Anaemia

- Mild anaemia is a common late finding after gastrectomy. A haemoglobin of <10 g/dl and anaemia occurring less than 5 years after gastrectomy requires further investigation.
- Common causes include poor dietary intake of haematinics and bleeding from a recurrent ulcer or carcinoma. Malabsorption of iron should only be considered after bleeding from a colonic lesion has been excluded.
- Vitamin B_{12} deficiency after a partial gastrectomy (usually presenting as macrocytosis) is usually due to bacterial overgrowth, terminal ileum disease or pernicious anaemia, since enough parietal cells usually remain after a partial gastrectomy to produce sufficient intrinsic factor.

Cancer in gastric remnant

Controversy exists about the exact incidence of gastric cancer after a partial gastrectomy, but it has been estimated as 2.2 times that of controls 15 years after surgery. The risk seems greater after gastric ulcer, rather than duodenal ulcer, surgery, and after Billroth II, rather than Billroth I, procedures. Postoperative endoscopic surveillance is not indicated unless new symptoms arise.

Retained antrum

This is a very rare cause of recurrent ulceration and hypergastrinaemia. The diagnosis is made after excluding the Zollinger–Ellison syndrome.

Further reading

Eagon JC, Miedema BW, Kelly KA. Postgastrectomy syndromes. *Surgical Clinics of North America*, 1992; **72**: 445–65.

Thirlby RC. Evaluation of patients with postsurgical syndromes. *Gastroenterology Clinics of North America*, 1994; **23**: 189–92.

Tovey FI, Hall ML, Ell PJ, Hobsley M. A review of postgastrectomy bone disease. *Journal Gastroenterology and Hepatology*, 1992; **7**: 639–45.

Related topics of interest

PRIMARY BILIARY CIRRHOSIS

PBC is an autoimmune disease of unknown cause, characterized by the progressive destruction of small interlobular bile ducts by a chronic granulomatous inflammation, which results in cirrhosis. The prevalence varies widely between and within different countries (between 20 and 240 cases per 1 000 000 population). The incidence appears to be increasing, particularly in north-east England. It may present in any age (except childhood), and there is a family predisposition.

Clinical features

1. Symptoms. Ninety percent of patients are female, and the mean age at presentation is 60–70 years old. Up to 60% may be asymptomatic or present with fatigue only. The diagnosis is often made after finding an incidentally elevated ALP, or positive AMA during investigations for an associated condition (see below). The commonest symptom is the insidious onset of pruritus, frequently with malaise and sometimes right-upper quadrant discomfort. Pruritus may start during pregnancy. Jaundice usually develops between 6 months and 2 years after the onset of pruritus.

2. Examination. During the early stages, the patient is well nourished and may have generalized hyperpigmentation, scratch marks and hepatosplenomegaly. Oesophageal varices (and bleeding from them) may develop before other signs of chronic liver disease, which only occur in the very late stages. Xanthelasma and xanthoma are common findings in the latter stages of the disease, and often disappear in the terminal stages. Osteoporosis and osteomalacia presenting as pathological fractures and bone pain are common, particularly in those with marked cholestasis. Other features of fat-soluble vitamin malabsorption include night blindness (hypovitaminosis A) and easy bruising (vitamin K deficiency).

Associated conditions

Autoimmune diseases are found in up to 80% of patients, and almost any autoimmune disease has been associated. The sicca syndrome occurs in about 80% and the following are also frequently found:

- Thyroiditis.
- CD.
- Dermatomyositis.
- Mixed connective tissue disease.
- Rheumatoid arthritis.
- Raynaud's syndrome.
- Fibrosing alveolitis.
- Sclerodactyly.
- SLE.

There is a greater than expected incidence of inflammatory bowel disease. Finger clubbing is common and may be associated with hypertrophic osteoarthropathy.

Laboratory investigations Serum ALP, GGT and bilirubin are raised – the latter is seldom >35 μmol/l except in the late stages. Serum IgM is often raised. Synthetic liver function is retained in the early stages. Fat-soluble vitamin deficiencies may arise secondary to cholestasis in the later stages. Hypercholesterolaemia is common; levels fall as the disease progresses.

Diagnosis *1. Anti-mitochondrial antibody.* AMA is found in 90–95% of patients and anti-nuclear antibodies in approximately a quarter. Subspecies of AMA are also found in drug-induced diseases, SLE and various infections (including CMV infection). The M2 subtype is specific for PBC. Autoimmune cholangitis is the term used for the small number of patients with histological features of PBC, but absent AMA. The clinical course and response to treatment is the same as for PBC.

2. Liver biopsy. A liver biopsy is routinely used to confirm the diagnosis and four histological grades of disease are recognized:

- Stage I: Florid bile duct lesions with shrunken and vacuolated bile duct cells surrounded by granulomatous lesions.
- Stage II: Spread of inflammation out of the portal triads with biliary piecemeal necrosis.
- Stage III: Scarring (septal fibrosis and bridging).
- Stage IV: Cirrhosis.

The practice of performing a liver biopsy routinely is, however, debatable as the presence of M2 AMA is in itself virtually diagnostic, and histological changes do not have a bearing on prognosis. Furthermore, changes in the liver are focal and evolve at different speeds in different parts. Similar changes may also be seen in sarcoidosis, graft-versus-host disease, hepatitis C and, rarely, secondary biliary cirrhosis.

Course and prognosis
- The rate of progression of disease is very variable between patients. In general:
  Asymptomatic patients diagnosed with an abnormal ALP and AMA have a median time from diagnosis to death of 8–12 years. This is likely to be much longer as cases are now being detected at a much earlier asymptomatic stage than previously.
  Patients who present with symptoms of pruritus and lethargy have a median time to transplantation or death of 5–10 years.

Those patients with signs of liver decompensation (e.g. jaundice, ascites, malnutrition) have a median time to death or transplantation of 3–5 years.

Patients with a serum bilirubin of >100 μmol/l are unlikely to survive >2 years.

- An accurate assessment of prognosis is important so as to determine the optimum time for liver transplantation. Although prognostic models cannot be entirely accurate, the best validated is the Mayo Clinic prognostic model. This is based on variables of age, serum bilirubin, serum albumin, PT and oedema, used in a formula to estimate the survival probability at any given time.
- Up to 50% of men may die from a hepatoma. Women have a greatly increased relative risk of developing a hepatoma, but this is still rare.

Treatment

1. *General and symptomatic*

(a) Pruritus

- Cholestyramine (a bile acid-binding resin), at a dose of 4 g before and after breakfast, and if necessary before the midday and evening meal, is effective in most patients. Adverse effects are frequent and include bloating, diarrhoea, nausea and drug- and fat-soluble vitamin malabsorption.
- Rifampicin (a hepatic enzyme inducer) is the only other proven effective treatment.
- Ursodeoxycholic acid (UDCA), phenobarbitone, opioid-receptor antagonists, stanazol, PUVA and plasmapharesis have been tried in resistant cases, but their efficacy is unproven.
- Antihistamines are useful only for their sedative effect, and should generally be avoided.

(b) Lethargy

- This is present in most patients and is the most debilitating symptom in half of patients.
- It is important to exclude other, treatable causes such as thyroid disease, adrenal insufficiency and medication adverse effects.
- The serotonin-1A receptor agonist, buspirone, is currently being evaluated as treatment.

(c) Nutrition

- Dietary advice should be obtained to maintain an adequate caloric and protein intake.
- Medium-chain triglyceride supplements are used for those with steatorrhoea.
- Vitamins K, A, E and D should be replaced as necessary. The route of administration depends on the severity of deficiency and disease – parenteral supplements are needed when cholestasis occurs (as evinced by a rising bilirubin).

(d) Bone disease
- Osteoporosis is a significant problem. It is due to malabsorption of calcium, use of corticosteroids and possibly also a direct toxic effect of bilirubin.
- A daily intake of 1.5 g of calcium should be aimed at, exercise and safe sunlight exposures encouraged and hormone replacement therapy should be considered for postmenopausal patients.
- Cyclical bisphosphonates with calcium are unproven but may be beneficial.
- The response to treatment may be monitored with bone densitometry scans.
- Osteomalacia is less common and is due to vitamin D malabsorption. Ideally, vitamin D levels should be monitored and 1,25–dihydroxy-D$_3$ replacement given parenterally in cholestasis.

2. *Disease-modifying treatment*
(a) Ursodeoxycholic acid
- UDCA is a naturally occurring bile acid which is currently the only agent licensed specifically for the treatment of PBC.
- It improves liver biochemistry and leads to a fall in the AMA titre and Ig levels. It leads to a modest reduction in the development and progression of portal hypertension and prolongs survival and time to transplant.
- Symptomatic patients should be treated with a single daily dose of 10–15 mg/kg. It is usually well tolerated, with diarrhoea being the only significant adverse effect. This can usually be ameliorated by reducing or splitting the dose.
(b) Other agents
- Cyclosporin A reduces symptoms and may prolong survival, but side-effects including hypertension and nephrotoxicity preclude its routine use.
- Methotrexate, azathioprine and tacrolimus all remain experimental, but are potentially beneficial.
- Colchicine improves liver function but has no effect on survival, and is rarely used due to a high incidence of side-effects.

3. *Liver transplantation.* Liver transplantation should be considered in the following circumstances:

- Prognostic markers indicate a survival of <1 year.
- Biochemistry shows a falling serum albumin (<30 g/l) or increasing bilirubin (>150 μmol/l).
- Uncontrollable complications (e.g. ascites, bleeding oesophageal varices, encephalopathy, recurrent sponta-

neous bacterial peritonitis, progressive muscle wasting, worsening osteoporosis).
- Intractable symptoms (e.g. pruritus, lethargy).

The 5-year survival after transplant is about 80%. Twenty-five percent will need a re-transplant due to recurrence of disease in the graft.

Further reading

Neuberger J. Primary biliary cirrhosis. *Lancet*, 1997; **350**: 875–9.

Related topics of interest

PRIMARY SCLEROSING CHOLANGITIS

- PSC is an idiopathic syndrome of progressive inflammation and fibrosis of the intra- and/or extrahepatic biliary tree resulting in chronic cholestasis.
- The condition is associated with ulcerative colitis in 75% of cases. Symptoms of ulcerative colitis may predate or antedate the diagnosis of PSC. The extent or activity of ulcerative colitis does not predict the course.
- It is to be distinguished from secondary sclerosing cholangitis which may be caused by the following:
  Recurrent choledocholithiasis.
  Traumatic stricture post-ERCP or surgery.
  Diffuse cholangiocarcinoma.
  Infections (e.g. *Cryptococcus*, *Cryptosporidium* or CMV infection in AIDS patients).
  Congenital anomalies.
- The aetiology of PSC is unknown, but it is thought to be an autoimmune disease possibly triggered by a transient biliary tract infection.

Clinical features

- Seventy percent of patients are male and most present in the fourth or fifth decade.
- A common mode of presentation is asymptomatic elevation of ALP in a patient with ulcerative colitis (or, rarely, colonic Crohn's disease). The ulcerative colitis usually affects the whole large bowel and is quiescent at the time of presentation.
- The gradual progression of fatigue, pruritus and obstructive jaundice are common clinical features. Rarely, patients may present with episodes of clinical cholangitis or features of chronic liver disease (e.g. ascites, variceal bleeding).

Complications

- Cholangiocarcinoma develops in 10–15% of cases of PSC, and is commonest in those with long-standing ulcerative colitis. The diagnosis is notoriously difficult to make in the early stages, when it is potentially treatable. Suggestive features at ERCP include a progressive biliary stricture with localized proximal dilatation, and intraductal polyps. Biopsies and/or brushings for cytology should be taken from any suspicious lesion. Serial measurement of serum tumour markers such as CA19-9 and CEA may help in the diagnosis.
- PSC is a risk factor for the development of colonic dysplasia and colorectal carcinoma in those with ulcerative colitis, although the magnitude of this risk is debatable.
- Recurrent bacterial cholangitis is common during the course of the disease, particularly in those with common bile duct strictures.

- Cholelithiasis and choledocholithiasis occur in up to 30% of cases owing to prolonged biliary stasis.
- Dominant extrahepatic strictures develop at some stage of the disease in 15–20% of patients.

Investigations

- ERCP is the method of choice for diagnosis. The usual finding is of diffuse, multiple strictures with intervening dilatation ('beading') of the intrahepatic tree. One-third have strictures of the extrahepatic tree.
- Serum ALP is almost invariably raised. Serum transaminases and GGT are also commonly elevated.
- Unlike primary biliary cirrhosis, no serological markers exist, and autoantibody titres (including AMA) are usually normal.
- Liver ultrasound excludes other conditions which may mimic PSC (e.g. polycystic liver disease, metastasis, cholelithiasis).
- Liver biopsy is often characteristic and allows staging. The most frequent finding is a fibrous obliterative cholangitis with periductal lymphocytic infiltration. Similar findings may be found in PBC and chronic active hepatitis.

Treatment

1. *Disease-modifying treatment*
- Penicillamine, corticosteroids, azathioprine and colchicine have all been tried, but no medical therapy has been shown to be of benefit.
- UDCA, in doses used to treat PBC, has been shown to reduce liver enzymes, but does not affect survival. Trials are underway using larger doses in an attempt to prolong survival.
- Proctocolectomy does not alter the course of the disease in those with ulcerative colitis.
- Liver transplantation is the only effective treatment. The timing for transplantation is difficult, owing to the wide variability in the course of the disease. Several prognostic models have been devised to define this. The Mayo Clinic model uses the serum bilirubin level, histological stage and the presence of splenomegaly, but is not able to predict the development of cholangiocarcinoma. The 5-year survival after liver transplantation is approximately 50%. Strictures develop in the transplanted bile ducts more frequently than other transplant groups, and may be due to disease recurrence, ischaemia, infection or rejection.

2. *Complications specific to primary sclerosing cholangitis*
- Cholangitis is treated with i.v. antibiotics. Anecdotal reports have shown that prophylactic ciprofloxacin may prevent further attacks.

- Endoscopic treatment allows dilatation, stent insertion of dominant strictures, and removal of stones or biliary debris.

3. *Complications associated with chronic cholestatic liver disease*
- Pruritus may be severely debilitating and may be treated with cholestyramine (4–12 g/day) and/or chlorphenarimine (24 mg/day) for symptomatic relief.
- Steatorrhoea can be ameliorated with a low-fat diet, cholestyramine and codeine phosphate or imodium to reduce stool frequency.
- Fat-soluble vitamin malabsorption requires monthly i.m. injections of vitamin K and vitamin A. Osteoporosis and osteomalacia are treated with 1-α-cholecalciferol (1 µg daily) and calcium (1.5 g daily), with the avoidance of corticosteroids.

The management of complications related to portal hypertension and hepatic encephalopathy are covered elsewhere.

Prognosis
- The average survival from the time of diagnosis is about 10 years in symptomatic patients. Asymptomatic patients have a better survival, possibly as long as 17 years.
- The cause of death is usually liver failure, variceal haemorrhage or cholangiocarcinoma.
- Those with intrahepatic duct involvement alone have a better prognosis than those with any extrahepatic duct involvement.

Further reading

Chapman RW. Aetiology and natural history of primary sclerosing cholangitis – a decade of progress? *Gut*, 1991; **32(12)**: 1433–5.

Related topics of interest

PSEUDOMEMBRANOUS COLITIS

Aetiology and pathogenesis

Pseudomembranous colitis (PMC) is caused by infection with the organism *Clostridium difficile* and is a common cause of diarrhoea in hospitalized and institutionalized patients. Most cases follow a course of antibiotics, usually broad-spectrum antibiotics that affect enteric organisms. This leads to disruption of the normal colonic bacterial flora and allows the colonization of *C. difficile*, which releases toxins (principally toxin A) that cause mucosal inflammation and damage. Infection with *C. difficile* occurs via the faecal–oral route, either from infected patients, contaminated surfaces in the hospital setting (heat-resistant spores are able to persist for years) or from asymptomatic carriers. Healthy adults are rarely carriers of *C. difficile*, but approximately 25% of adults who have recently been treated with antibiotics are colonized.

PMC represents the severe end of the spectrum of *C. difficile*-induced diarrhoea, and the organism is also a common cause of antibiotic-associated diarrhoea in the absence of PMC. In rare cases, PMC follows a course of chemotherapy. Antibiotics that are associated with PMC are listed below.

- Those that frequently induce PMC are cephalosporins, augmentin, amoxicillin, ampicillin and clindamycin (the latter causes diarrhoea in 10% of patients and PMC in 1%).
- Those that infrequently induce PMC are erythromycin, trimethoprim, tetracyclines and quinolones.
- Those that rarely or never induce PMC are metronidazole, vancomycin and i.v. aminoglycosides.

Clinical features

- *C. difficile* infection most often presents as watery diarrhoea which usually occurs during or shortly after a course of antibiotics; the symptoms may, however, be delayed for several weeks. Systemic features are absent, and the diarrhoea usually abates after withdrawal of the antibiotic. The diagnosis is made by the finding of *C. difficile* toxin in the stool, and a sigmoidoscopy, although not essential, will be normal.
- PMC presents with profuse watery or bloody diarrhoea, abdominal discomfort, bloating, fever, anorexia and nausea. A sigmoidoscopy will reveal characteristic yellowish plaques ('pseudomembranes') which vary in size from 2–10 mm, or coalesce to cover large areas. The intervening mucosa is usually only mildly erythematous. The features are most prominent in the rectosigmoid, but may extend, or predominantly affect, the descending colon.

- In rare cases, patients present with an acute abdomen and fulminant colitis. Toxic dilatation of the colon may occur (as in acute ulcerative colitis), which results in a paradoxical decrease in diarrhoea. An abdominal radiograph will show colonic dilatation and mucosal oedema ('thumb printing'), and if a perforation has occurred, free air will be seen under the diaphragm on a chest radiograph. A sigmoidoscopy should be avoided in fulminant colitis because of the risk of perforation, but a careful limited proctoscopy may be performed to confirm the diagnosis.

Diagnostic investigations

- A stool specimen should be sent for *C. difficile* toxin testing. The stool cytotoxin test has a sensitivity and specificity that approaches 100%; however, it is expensive and requires overnight incubation. Enzyme immunoassays are quicker, cheaper and easier to perform, but are not as sensitive. It is therefore worth sending more than one stool specimen for analysis.
- Stool cultures for *C. difficile* are not routinely performed as this leads to a delay in the diagnosis and non-toxigenic commensal strains may be isolated.
- The pathognomonic histological feature is a prominent exudate extending from an area of epithelial ulceration ('volcano lesion'). This 'pseudomembrane' consists of fibrin, neutrophils and cellular debris. The intervening mucosa is normal or only mildly inflamed.

Differential diagnosis

Acute ulcerative colitis may be difficult to distinguish histologically from mild cases of PMC. In elderly patients, acute ischaemic colitis may mimic the clinical features of PMC. In both cases, a stool toxin assay will be discriminatory.

Treatment

- Existing antibiotic treatment must be discontinued.
- Oral metronidazole (250 mg four times daily) or oral vancomycin (125 mg four times daily) are equally effective. Symptomatic improvement usually occurs within 72 hours, and most patients respond completely after 10 days of treatment. Although metronidazole is more likely to cause adverse effects (e.g. nausea, metallic taste in the mouth and disulfiram-like reactions), it is the agent of first choice as it is significantly less expensive than vancomycin. Metronidazole (but not vancomycin) is also effective when given intravenously.
- Patients are often advised to consume natural yoghurt, but this has not been shown to be beneficial.
- Fulminant colitis and toxic dilatation should be treated with a 48–72 hour trial of i.v. metronidazole with the necessary supportive treatment and close monitoring. A sub-

total colectomy should be considered if there has been no improvement after this time.

Management of relapse   Up to 30% of patients have a relapse of diarrhoea within 1–3 weeks after treatment has been discontinued. This is either due to a failure to eradicate the organism, or to re-infection. The diagnosis is confirmed by a stool toxin assay. Mild relapses usually settle spontaneously in the absence of further treatment, which makes a subsequent relapse less likely. More severe or persistent relapses of diarrhoea should be treated with a second course of metronidazole (or vancomycin if metronidazole has not been tolerated). Symptoms usually settle rapidly, but further relapses are not uncommon. These may be prevented by prolonged treatment over several weeks, and by reducing the dose gradually. Cholestyramine, rifampicin or the oral administration of non-toxigenic strains of *C. difficile* have been evaluated for resistant cases, but their efficacy is unproven.

Further reading

Kelly CP, Pothoulakis C, LaMont JT. *Clostridium difficile* colitis. *New England Journal of Medicine*, 1994; **330**: 62.

Related topics of interest

Colitis – non-specific (p. 50)
Ulcerative colitis – background and clinical features (p. 265)
Ulcerative colitis – medical and surgical management (p. 269)

RADIATION ENTERITIS

Radiation-induced damage to the gut occurs most frequently following radiotherapy for pelvic or abdominal malignancy. The amount of damage to the bowel depends upon the total cumulative dose of radiation (>4000 rads) and the size of the area irradiated. Previous abdominal surgery increases the risk because the bowel is often fixed by adhesions, thus subjecting the same loops of bowel to the field of irradiation. Both the small and large bowel may be affected, with the ileum being most susceptible. The damage mainly affects the submucosal layer, and hence is not always detected by routine biopsies. With time an endarteritis develops resulting in ischaemia. Patients may experience symptoms at the time of radiotherapy or at some later stage.

Acute radiation injury

- Transient diarrhoea or constipation is common during a course of radiotherapy and may be due to an ileus. It usually settles spontaneously and does not indicate permanent damage.
- Acute radiation enteritis produces nausea, abdominal cramps and watery diarrhoea (occasionally blood-stained).
- Acute proctocolitis presents with tenesmus, diarrhoea and a mucoid or bloody rectal discharge.
- Nausea and vomiting often follows upper abdominal radiotherapy and may be related to acute gastroparesis.
- In those with colorectal involvement, colonoscopy may show an oedematous inflamed mucosa, diffuse erythema, submucosal telangectasia (similar in appearance to those found on the abdominal skin), superficial ulceration or may appear normal.

Late radiation injury

- Late symptoms often develop insidiously after an asymptomatic period of up to 20 years. Some patients have a history of transient acute radiation enteritis, but others have no record of bowel radiation injury and the diagnosis may be overlooked, especially if symptoms develop some time after the initial radiotherapy. Many of the clinical and radiological features resemble Crohn's disease.
- In the small bowel, the ileum is most susceptible to radiation damage. The cardinal features are mucosal and submucosal inflammation and an endarteritis which results in intestinal ischaemia, ulceration, fibrosis, stricture formation and altered motility. Fistulae may form between the small and large bowel or to adjacent pelvic organs (e.g. bladder or vagina). Occasionally free perforation occurs, resulting in acute peritonitis.
- The splenic flexure, sigmoid and rectum are the most susceptible areas in the large bowel. Chronic inflammation, ulceration and fibrosis may produce strictures, fistulae and

pelvic abscesses. Discrete ulceration or strictures may be found in the rectum.

Clinical features

These may include:

- Colicky abdominal pain (partial or complete bowel obstruction due to strictures, adhesions or dysmotility).
- Watery diarrhoea (generalized mucosal damage, lactose intolerance due to brush border depletion or small bowel bacterial overgrowth due to fistulae, strictures or impaired motility).
- Steatorrhoea (bile salt malabsorption in the distal ileum).
- Tenesmus, mucoid or bloody rectal discharge (proctitis or rectal ulceration).

Investigations

- Barium contrast studies of the small bowel may show dilated, separated loops of hypotonic small bowel, mucosal oedema and excessive secretions in the lumen. Progressive fibrosis may produce a fixed, narrowed, featureless segment. Barium enema studies may show mucosal oedema ('thumb printing' which mimics intestinal ischaemia), fistulae or strictures (which may mimic a carcinoma). Late changes in the rectosigmoid include shortening, superficial ulceration and the loss of haustral folds, similar to ulcerative colitis.
- Depending on the stage of radiation change, colonoscopy may reveal an oedematous, granular, friable mucosa with multiple submucosal telangectasiae. Strictures and superficial or discrete ulceration may also be found.
- Histologically, a chronic transmural inflammatory infiltrate, ulceration and endarteritis is seen. The findings are often characteristic but may be confused with Crohn's disease.
- A CT scan is useful to detect the possible recurrence of a tumour and to clarify the findings of barium studies. Malabsorption studies are important for those with suggestive clinical or biochemical features. Lactose intolerance (disaccharidase deficiency due to brush border depletion) is diagnosed with a lactose breath hydrogen test. Bile acid malabsorption due to terminal ileum disease is detected with the SeHCAT test. Bacterial overgrowth due to strictures, fistulae or impaired motility can be diagnosed with the glucose (or lactulose) breath hydrogen test or glycocholate breath test.

Management

1. *Early symptoms*
- Acute symptoms during treatment usually settle with stopping or reducing the radiotherapy.
- Nausea can usually be controlled with a phenothiazine or dopamine antagonist and diarrhoea usually responds to antidiarrhoeal agents (e.g. imodium).

- A lactose-free diet may be helpful and cholestyramine (4–12 g/day) should be tried if bile salt malabsorption is likely.

2. *Late/chronic symptoms*
- Radiation proctitis or colitis sometimes responds to steroid retention enemas or 5-ASA tablets or enemas.
- Diarrhoea should be investigated and the cause treated: bile salt malabsorption with a low-fat diet and cholestyramine; lactose intolerance with a lactose-free diet; bacterial overgrowth with broad-spectrum antibiotics.
- Nutritional supplementation with medium-chain triglycerides, polymeric or monomeric diets may be useful in those with probable dysmotility. For those patients with generalized small bowel involvement and who respond poorly to treatment, total parenteral nutrition can provide a marked improvement.
- Rectal bleeding from colonic telangectasiae may be controlled with bipolar electrocoagulation or laser photocoagulation.
- Certain colonic or rectal strictures may be dilated with transendoscopic balloon dilatation.
- Surgery is indicated for the excision of large strictures or fistulae; however, the complication rate is high and healing is generally poor.

Further reading

Muller AF. Physico-chemical trauma to the gut. *Medicine International*, 1994; **22**: 353–8.

Related topics of interest

Diarrhoea (p. 81)
Malabsorption (p. 189)

RECTAL BLEEDING

Bleeding from the lower gastrointestinal tract is characterized by the passage of fresh or maroon-coloured blood per rectum. It can usually be distinguished from UGT bleeding, which results in black, tarry stools (melaena).

Causes of lower gastrointestinal bleeding

Small intestine

1. Meckel's diverticulum. This occurs in 2% of the population and lies in the last 90 cm of the ileum. It occurs equally in both sexes, and can present at any age, but usually presents in boys in childhood or the early teenage years. Most present with the single or recurrent passage of bright red or maroon bleeding per rectum, or less frequently with an iron deficiency anaemia. The diverticulum may contain heterotrophic gastric epithelium, and bleeding is from peptic ulceration in the neck of the diverticulum. The diagnosis can be made with a sodium pertechnetate isotope (Meckel's) scan (if the diverticulum contains ectopic gastric tissue), barium small bowel series, or selective superior mesenteric angiogram. Surgical wedge resection is the treatment of choice.

2. Crohn's disease. Rectal bleeding is less common with Crohn's disease than with ulcerative colitis. Ileal Crohn's disease is a relatively frequent cause of acute rectal bleeding in younger patients, but is a rare cause in adults.

3. Other causes
- Arteriovenous malformation.
- Angiodysplasia.
- Polyps.
- Jejunal diverticulae.
- Tumours (e.g. carcinoma, lymphoma, leiomyoma, Kaposi's sarcoma).
- Mesenteric ischaemia.
- Tuberculosis.
- Postsurgical anastomotic ulcer.

Colon and rectum

1. Angiodysplasia. This is an important cause of acute, chronic and occult lower gastrointestinal bleeding. These occur mainly in the right colon and caecum, and the incidence increases with age. They are described as small collections of mucosal and submucosal ectatic vessels, usually on the antimesenteric surface. An association with aortic stenosis and chronic obstructive airways disease is described, but the aetiology is uncertain.

2. Other causes (many of these are discussed elsewhere)
- Diverticular disease.
- Arteriovenous malformations.
- Ischaemic colitis.
- Polyps.
- Colorectal carcinoma.
- Ulcerative colitis.
- Crohn's disease.
- Peri-anal conditions (e.g. fissures, haemorrhoids).
- Solitary rectal ulcer.
- Ano-rectal varices (secondary to portal hypertension).
- Postoperative (e.g. postpolypectomy, anastomotic ulcer).
- Radiation proctitis or enteritis.

Management approach

1. Assessment of severity. The description of the amount of bleeding, pulse, blood pressure (including postural drop), rectal examination and blood tests (full blood count, coagulation screen, electrolytes, cross-match) are all important. Urgent resuscitation is needed for those with severe bleeding. A central venous line will be needed in such cases, and is useful to monitor further transfusion requirements.

2. Establish the site and cause of bleeding. A rigid sigmoidoscopy is a useful initial investigation and will detect local lesions. Further investigations depend on whether the bleeding subsides or not, and on the severity of bleeding.

3. Investigations for ongoing bleeding. Colonoscopy or flexible sigmoidoscopy may not be successful initially, due to poor visibility, and are ideally performed following a suitable bowel preparation (e.g. oral polyethylene glycol or phosphate enema). Good views of the right colon should be achieved, as angiodysplasia is commonest in this region, and is easily overlooked. Using a large-channel instrument to provide adequate suction, experienced endoscopists are able to detect the exact site of bleeding in 50% of such cases, and the region of bleeding in 70%. In addition, diffuse bleeding from colitis may be evident.

An upper gastrointestinal endoscopy may be necessary if the above do not clearly define the site of bleeding. A radionuclide scan may detect extravasation of blood into the bowel lumen when the rate of haemorrhage is as low as 0.5–1 ml/min. It is also able to detect the anatomical lesion accounting for the bleeding (e.g. eroding aneurysm or tumour). Colloid radionuclide scanning, which involves the i.v. administration of ^{99m}Tc-labelled sulphur colloid, is best in the acute setting. Regional localization of bleeding is usually only possible, however. Red blood cell radionuclide scanning involves the injection of

^{99m}Tc-*in vitro*-labelled autologous red blood cells. This method provides better images, but is more time consuming.

Selective mesenteric angiography is a valuable investigation if the bleeding rate exceeds 0.5 ml/min. It is, however, technically demanding and ideally should only be performed by experienced radiologists, as prolonged procedures may delay adequate resuscitation and definitive treatment.

A barium enema or small bowel series are indicated to detect structural lesions if the above tests are inconclusive.

Laparotomy and on-table examination of the bowel digitally and endoscopically are required in some cases. A further technique for localizing the general area of gastrointestinal bleeding in recurrent cases is to isolate small/large bowel or right/left colon by use of ileostomy/colostomy, and observe which orifice bleeds. Endoscopy via such 'ostomies' may be of use.

4. Investigations for bleeding which has spontaneously stopped. A colonoscopy following adequate bowel preparation gives the greatest diagnostic yield. A selective mesenteric angiogram may detect mucosal vascular lesions. A barium enema or small bowel series may give additional information.

Treatment of severe bleeding

1. Non-surgical
- After resuscitation, the definitive treatment depends upon the cause of bleeding.
- Although correction of a coagulation abnormality may be therapeutic, the source of bleeding in such cases should still be sought and treated appropriately.
- Definitive colonoscopic procedures include snare polypectomy for bleeding polyps; adrenaline injection or laser coagulation for bleeding tumours or arteriovenous malformations; and electrocoagulation or laser ablation for angiodysplasia.
- When a site of bleeding has been identified by angiography, the selective infusion of vasopressin may be beneficial, but often only temporarily.
- Arteriographic embolization is an option when the site of haemorrhage has been localized by angiography. Bowel ischaemia is a recognized complication, and this should only be considered by experienced operators, and in patients who are unable to tolerate a surgical procedure.

2. Surgery
- When a bleeding source is identified by the above investigations, segmental resection is the operation of choice.
- A laparotomy should always be considered when the blood transfusion requirements excede 6 units.

- With the increased use of angiography and on-table enteroscopy, blind right or left colectomy should rarely be needed nowadays.
- If such measures are required (i.e. for persistent bleeding), the nature of the blood loss is a rough guide to the origin of the bleeding. Melaena-like stools usually arise from angiodysplasia (or, less commonly, diverticulae) in the proximal colon, which is relatively common in the elderly, while fresh bleeding usually arises from the left colon (often secondary to diverticulosis). The rule is by no means fallible, and if uncertainty exists, a blind right hemicolectomy is a reasonable procedure if the patient is elderly and continues to bleed.

Prognosis   Although 85% of lower gastrointestinal bleeds stop spontaneously, the overall mortality is about 10%. This reflects the fact that most acute lower gastrointestinal bleeds occur in the elderly, who tolerate surgery poorly (the mortality for acute colonic surgery in the elderly is about 50%).

Further reading

Raine PA. Investigation of rectal bleeding. *Archives of Disease in Childhood*, 1991; **66(3)**: 279–80.

Related topic of interest

Haematemesis and melaena (p. 135)

SMALL BOWEL DIVERTICULOSIS

Duodenal diverticula

True duodenal diverticula are usually found incidentally and do not cause any symptoms. They often occur near the ampulla of Vater, and may impede access to the ampulla during an ERCP. 'Pseudodiverticula' are acquired as a result of previous duodenal ulceration, and are thus usually found in the duodenal bulb.

Duodenal diverticula occasionally cause the following complications:

- Bacterial proliferation in a diverticulum adjacent to the ampulla of Vater may lead to an ascending cholangitis and pancreatitis.
- The incidence of common bile duct stones is said to be higher in those with juxtapapillary diverticula, presumably due to biliary stasis.
- Bleeding and diverticulitis due to enterolith formation.

The treatment for recurring symptoms is surgical diverticulectomy, but is seldom necessary.

Jejunal diverticulosis

Jejunal diverticulosis is rare, with an estimated prevalence of 0.2–0.5%. The diverticula usually develop in the sixth or seventh decades, and less than half of patients ever become symptomatic. Most cases present from the seventh decade onwards; symptoms are non-specific, e.g. postprandial abdominal pain, nausea, fatty-food intolerance, bloating and change in bowel habit.

Complications
- Bacterial overgrowth and malabsorption occur in about 10% of cases. Deficiencies of fat-soluble vitamins (A, D, E and K), iron, magnesium and trace metals occur. Intestinal bacteria consume vitamin B_{12} and serum levels may be low, whereas they produce folate, serum levels of which may be high.
- Mechanical obstruction may occur *de novo* or as a result of a diverticular volvulus, faecolith, intussusception, adhesions or diverticulitis.
- Chronic small-bowel pseudo-obstruction is a relatively common problem and is probably due to jejunal dyskinesia.
- Acute diverticulitis and perforation is a rare but well described complication. Symptoms may simulate almost any other cause of an acute abdomen.
- Acute, fresh or altered rectal bleeding from one of the diverticula occurs in 4–5% of cases. Preoperative diagnosis is often difficult and may be helped by a radionucleotide red blood cell scan or mesenteric angiography.

Diagnosis	Enteroclysis of the small bowel is the investigation of choice in suspected cases. Plain abdominal radiography is usually unhelpful. Contrast-enhanced abdominal CT may show inflammatory changes in acute diverticulitis.

Treatment

- Bacterial overgrowth is treated with rotating courses of antibiotics – usually tetracycline and metronidazole.
- Nutritional deficiencies should be corrected.
- Some patients have an associated pancreatic exocrine deficiency, and require appropriate supplements.
- Those with jejunal dyskinesia may benefit from the cautious introduction of a prokinetic agent (e.g. cisapride).
- Surgical resection is seldom performed due to the diffuse nature of the disease. Complications (i.e. perforation or uncontrollable haemorrhage) are treated with surgical resection of the involved segment.

Meckel's diverticulum

This is an embryological remnant of the vitello-intestinal duct and is present in 2% of the population. It is usually situated 50 cm from the ileocaecal valve, may be of varying length and may be associated with other congenital abnormalities. Less than 5% produce symptoms due to complications (half of all complications occur in infants less than a year old).

Complications

- Haemorrhage. This is more common than in other small bowel diverticula, as about 20% have ectopic gastric mucosa which is prone to ulceration. It is the most common mode of presentation in infants, and characteristically produces painless bright red or maroon bleeding (although it may be occult).
- Diverticulitis and perforation. Diverticulitis mimics acute appendicitis, and if associated with a band, obstruction may coexist. Perforation occurs in 15% and is potentially life-threatening.
- Other complications. Bacterial overgrowth, intussusception, volvulus and incarceration into an indirect inguinal (Littre's) hernia may rarely occur.

Diagnosis

- The diagnosis is frequently difficult and is often made at laparotomy.
- Small-bowel barium studies may be useful in adults, but are unhelpful in children.
- A technecium-99m pertechnetate isotope scan detects the presence of ectopic gastric mucosa, and may be useful in cases of bleeding. The sensitivity is increased by the addition of pentagastrin and glucagon.

Treatment	Complications are treated by surgical excision of the diverticulum and adjacent small bowel. Treatment of an incidental Meckel's diverticulum is contentious, but large diverticula should probably be surgically removed.

Further reading

Sibille A, Willcox R. Jejunal diverticulosis. *American Journal of Gastroenterology*, 1992; **87**: 655–8.

Related topics of interest

Malabsorption (p. 189)
Rectal bleeding (p. 247)

TRANSPLANTATION – LIVER

The number of patients eligible for, and receiving, liver transplants is increasing yearly. With little change in the number of donors, waiting lists extend and an examination of the selection criteria becomes necessary. The 1-year survival for elective transplants in low-risk patients is now approximately 90%. This level has been reached due to improvements in patient selection, surgical techniques, postoperative care, immunosuppressant regimens, and a greater tendency to re-transplant in the event of complications.

Patient selection

The timing of transplantation is often difficult. A broad consensus has been reached on the timing of transplant for end-stage chronic liver disease. These include a prothrombin ratio of >5, a serum albumin of <30 g/l, intractible ascites and bleeding oesophageal varices despite medical therapy. The indications and timing of transplant in PBC and ALF are outlined in the appropriate topics.

Conditions treated with liver transplantation

1. Cirrhosis. This remains the commonest indication with an overall 2-year survival of 75%; aetiological subtypes include:

(a) Viral hepatitis
- Hepatitis B. The 2-year survival is only 50–60% due to extrahepatic viral replication infecting the graft. Generally, only those patients who are HBV DNA- and hepatitis B 'e' antigen (HBeAg)-negative are candidates; however, successful transplantation has been described in HBV-positive cases using pre- and post-transplant antiviral therapies (e.g. lamivudine). Hepatitis B hyperimmune globulin has also been used to prevent graft re-infection.
- Hepatitis C. This is an increasing indication for liver transplantation (approximately one-third of all patients). Re-infection is almost invariable, and results in a mild chronic hepatitis. The 2-year survival is about 90%.
- Hepatitis D. Although re-infection of the graft is the rule, this inhibits hepatitis B recurrence and the 2-year survival is good (70%).

(b) Autoimmune chronic hepatitis
The disease does not recur post-transplant in most patients.

(c) Cryptogenic cirrhosis

(d) Alcoholic liver disease
This accounts for most cases of end-stage liver disease with cirrhosis in the West. Post-transplant survival is similar to that of other causes of cirrhosis, but at least 20% of patients resume alcohol after transplantation. The criteria for selection are contentious. These are:

- Abstinence from alcohol for 6 months.
- Child's grade C cirrhosis.

- Absence of extrahepatic organ alcohol damage.
- Stable socio-economic background (i.e. adequate family support) with a job to return to after the operation.

2. Malignant disease. Although this is the second most common indication at present, rates are reducing. Operative mortality is low, but long-term survival is poor (mostly due to carcinomatosis induced by immunosuppression). The 2-year survival is about 30%.

- Hepatocellular carcinoma. Indications are: single tumours of <5 cm which cannot be resected; or fewer than three multifocal tumours of <3 cm.
- Fibrolamellar carcinoma. These are not associated with cirrhosis, metastasize late and therefore have a better prognosis.

3. Cholestatic liver disease
- PBC. Prognosis is good with a 5-year survival of 70%. The disease may recur in the transplanted liver over time.
- PSC. Surgery is often difficult due to coexisting infective cholangitis, previous surgery and an increased incidence of cholangiocarcinoma. Recurrent bile duct strictures develop in the transplanted liver; causes include recurrent disease, ischaemia, rejection and infection. The 5-year survival is 60%.

4. Fulminant liver failure. This indication is becoming more common. Diseases include fulminant viral hepatitis, paracetamol overdose, adverse drug reactions, fatty liver of pregnancy and Wilson's disease. See also 'Acute liver failure' (p. 8).

5. Metabolic disorders. A number of inborn errors of metabolism occurring in childhood are effectively treated with liver transplantation. These diseases are either associated with progressive liver disease (e.g. α_1-antitrypsin deficiency, galactosaemia, glycogen storage diseases, tyrosinaemia, cystic fibrosis) or cause predominantly extrahepatic complications due to enzyme defects (e.g. oxaluria, homozygous hypercholesterolaemia, Crigler–Najjar syndrome). The overall 5-year survival is 85%.

6. Miscellaneous
- Budd–Chiari syndrome.
- Short-bowel syndrome resulting in secondary liver failure; a combined small bowel and liver transplantation is performed.

Contraindications

1. Absolute contraindications
- Active sepsis.

- Metastatic malignancy.
- Uncorrectable cardiopulmonary disease.
- AIDS.
- Psychosocial factors.

2. *Factors associated with a high perioperative risk*
- Age <2 or >60.
- Previous hepatobiliary surgery.
- Portal vein thrombosis.
- Multiple organ transplants.
- Creatinine >2 mg/dl.
- Re-transplant.
- CMV mismatch.
- Advanced liver disease (particularly if being artificially ventilated).
- Other organ failure (e.g. cardiac, respiratory).

Preoperative preparation Blood group, HLA and DR antigens are recorded. The hepatic arteries, portal vessels and biliary tree are all imaged. Vaccines against hepatitis B, influenza and pneumococcus should be given. Blood should be collected for autologous transfusion later. All patients should receive psychological counselling and an explanation of the procedure and consequences.

New operative techniques
- Split liver grafts. Because of the shortage of available donors, an adult donor liver may be divided to provide two viable grafts. This technique is used in most paediatric transplants.
- Living-relative transplant. The left lateral segment of a liver from a living relative is sometimes used, usually for children with terminal disease and no suitable cadaveric grafts.
- Auxiliary partial liver transplantation. Part of the native liver is replaced by an equivalent portion of a donor liver. This technique has been used in ALF (when there is a chance that the host liver will spontaneously regenerate, thus precluding the need for long-term immunosuppression) and for certain metabolic diseases.

Immunosuppression
- Most centres use a combination of cyclosporin (or tacrolimus), azathioprine and corticosteroids to prevent graft rejection. The exact regimen and duration of immunosuppression is contentious.
- Cyclosporin has a narrow therapeutic index and levels need to be checked regularly. The major adverse effects are:
  Nephrotoxicity (enhanced by aminoglycosides).
  Hypertension.
  Hyperkalaemia.

Hypomagnesaemia.

Neurotoxicity (particularly those with a low serum cholesterol).

Weight gain.

Lymphoproliferative diseases.

Effects of immunosuppression.

- Azathioprine may cause myelosuppression, cholestasis, hepatitis and pancreatitis.
- Tacrolimus (FK506) is a new fungal extract similar to, but more potent than, cyclosporin. It is usually used to treat refractory rejection, but is the immunosuppressant agent of first choice in some centres.
- Monoclonal antibodies (against lymphocytes, CD3 receptor and interleukin-2 (IL-2) receptor) are currently being evaluated and show promise.

Post-transplant complications

Re-transplantation is required in 20–25% of patients, principally due to primary graft failure, hepatic artery thrombosis, chronic rejection and CMV infection. Postoperative complications can be divided into four broad categories.

1. Primary graft failure
- This occurs within the first 2 days and affects <5% of patients. It is due to inadequate donor liver preservation and the only treatment is re-transplantation.
- Technical complications related to surgery, hepatic artery thrombosis, portal vein thrombosis and respiratory, renal and CNS complications all contribute to postoperative morbidity and mortality.

2. Infections
- Infections complicate more than half of liver transplants. They may be primary, reactivation or opportunistic.
- Primary infection in the form of postoperative bacterial sepsis may be endogenous (from gut flora) or nosocomial. Primary CMV infection from the donor liver may occur.
- CMV reactivation occurs 4–6 weeks following most transplantation. It is the commonest cause of post-transplant hepatitis and, if it becomes chronic, is an indication for re-transplant. Postoperative gancyclovir is an effective prophylaxis. Reactivation of herpes simplex virus in the graft is effectively prevented with prophylactic acyclovir.
- Common opportunistic infections are *Pneumocystis carinii* (effectively prevented with cotrimoxazole for 6 months post-transplant) and fungal infections (particularly *Candida*).

3. *Graft rejection*
- Acute cellular rejection occurs between 5 and 30 days post-transplant. The diagnosis is confirmed with a liver biopsy and most cases are successfully treated by increased immunosuppression.
- Chronic ductopenic rejection presents as progressive cholestasis, usually within the first 3 months. The only treatment is re-transplantation.

4. *Biliary strictures.* These require ERCP assessment and stenting or balloon dilatation.

Further reading

Anon. Consensus statement on indications for liver transplantation: Paris, June 22–23. *Hepatology*, 1994; **20**: 635–685

McNair ANB, Tibbs CJ, Williams R. Hepatology. *British Medical Journal*, 1995; **311**: 1351–5.

O'Grady JG, Alexander GJ, Hayllar KM, Williams R. Early indicators of prognosis in fulminant hepatic failure. *Gastroenterology*, 1989; **97**: 439–45.

Shorrock C, Neuberger J. The changing face of liver transplantation. *Gut*, 1993; **34**: 295–8.

Related topics of interest

TRANSPLANTATION – SMALL BOWEL

- Small bowel transplantation (SBT) has become a potential alternative to long-term total parenteral nutrition (TPN) in patients with end-stage chronic intestinal failure.
- An estimated 2 per 1 000 000 people in the UK require SBT each year.
- The number of operations as well as the survival rates have improved significantly over the past decade, and the short-term survival rates are now on a par with those of lung transplantation.
- Most of the deaths after SBT are related to complications of immunosuppression. The recent introduction of tacrolimus has shown improved graft survival rates compared to cyclosporin.

Indications for small bowel transplantation

Intestinal failure is either due to loss of intestinal surface (i.e. short bowel syndrome) or a functional disturbance of gut motility and absorption. The main causes of intestinal failure treated with SBT are listed below:

1. *Infants and children*
- Necrotizing enterocolitis.
- Midgut volvulus.
- Gastroschisis.
- Microvillous inclusion disease.
- Visceral neuropathy.

2. *Adults*
- Massive surgical resection (from any cause).
- Crohn's disease.
- Small bowel infarction.
- Radiation injury.
- Strangulated hernia.
- Neoplasms (desmoid tumours).
- Chronic idiopathic pseudo-obstruction.

Long-term total parenteral nutrition

Home TPN has improved greatly since it was first introduced in the 1960s; however:

- It is inconvenient, expensive and long-term venous access is often difficult.
- Cholestatic liver disease and cirrhosis develop in some patients.
- It is associated with a number of social and psychological problems.

Despite the above, most children and adults on TPN do well.

Complications

- Several factors make the small intestine particularly difficult to transplant: the abundant amount of lymphoid tissue; the substantial quantity of microorganisms and the large

number of major histocompatability complex (MHC) antigens expressed on the surface of epithelial cells.
- Recognized complications include graft rejection (acute or chronic), sepsis (primary or related to immunosuppression), graft-versus-host disease or lymphoproliferative disease.

In order to become a routine treatment for intestinal failure, SBT must offer greater safety, lower costs and a better quality of life than TPN. Although considerable progress has been made, SBT cannot yet be considered a routine procedure to replace TPN.

Further reading

Asfar S, Zhong R, Grant D. Small bowel transplantation. *Surgical Clinics of North America*, 1994; **74(5)**: 1197–210.
Brousse N, Goulet O. Small bowel transplantation. *British Medical Journal*, 1996; **312**: 261–2.
Grant D. Current results of intestinal transplantation. *Lancet*, 1996; **347**: 1801–3.

Related topic of interest

Transplantation – liver (p. 254)

TUMOURS OF THE SMALL INTESTINE

Benign tumours

Leiomyomas

Leiomyomas are the commonest benign tumours of the small bowel. They usually present in middle age with occult bleeding. Treatment for those less than 5 cm in size is local excision; however, larger tumours need a wide excision as the risk of malignant transformation is increased.

Other forms of solitary polyps

- Adenomas occur sporadically or as part of the familial polyposis syndrome (see 'Hereditary neoplastic syndromes of the intestine' (p. 166)). Symptoms are unusual, but bleeding or intussusception may occur. Villous adenomas of the small intestine have a high incidence of malignant change (up to 50% in larger lesions). They are usually found in the duodenum and are best treated with segmental resection.
- Lipomas are usually found in males from the sixth decade onwards and occur most commonly in the ileum. They rarely produce symptoms (bleeding or obstruction) and never undergo malignant change. They produce characteristic features on barium studies and CT scan and uncomplicated lesions do not require removal.
- Lymphomas may occasionally present as a nodular polyp.

Multiple small bowel polyps

These are more common than single polyps.

- Nodular lymphoid hyperplasia occurs as multiple lymphoid aggregates in the ileum or rectum of children. They may be associated with hypogammaglobulinaemia.
- Non-neoplastic hamartomas of the small bowel are found as part of the Peutz–Jegher's syndrome (together with bucco-labial pigmentation).
- Multiple hamartomatous polyps are found in the duodenum (and occasionally in the stomach, colon and the rest of the small bowel) as part of the Cronkhite–Canada syndrome. The disease usually presents in childhood with malabsorption, alopecia, nail dystrophy and hypertrophied gastric folds.
- Neurofibromatosis and endometriosis are other causes of multiple benign small bowel polyps.

Malignant tumours

Adenocarcinomas

- Adenocarcinomas are the second most common malignant tumours of the small intestine (after carcinoid tumours).
- Most present between the ages of 50 and 80 with features of intermittent obstruction, bleeding and weight loss.
- Predisposing diseases include Crohn's disease, Peutz–Jegher's syndrome, CD and Gardener's syndrome.
- Most present as ulcerating areas in the duodenum and jejunum, and probably arise from pre-existing adenomatous polyps.
- Treatment is surgical resection; however, most adenocarcinomas have spread to the regional mesenteric lymph nodes by the time of diagnosis and are incurable.
- The overall 5-year survival rate is poor and ranges between 5 and 25%.

Small intestinal lymphomas

Primary extra-intestinal lymphomas (especially high-grade Burkitt's lymphoma) may spread to involve the intestine, but the manifestations and treatment are those of the primary disease. Primary small bowel lymphomas are uncommon, but after the stomach, they are the commonest site of extranodal lymphomas. These are divided into two types.

1. Western-type lymphomas. These account for 15% of small bowel malignancies and 28% of primary gut lymphomas. They are commoner in males and present either before 15 years of age, or in the fifth or sixth decades. Conditions predisposing to the development of small bowel lymphomas include CD, dermatitis herpetiformis, follicular lymphoid hyperplasia, inflammatory bowel disease, AIDS, and previous immunosuppressant therapy or radiotherapy.

(a) Features

- The tumour arises from gut-associated lymphoid tissue and thus has many features in common with primary lymphomas arising elsewhere in the gastrointestinal tract.
- Lesions may be large and polypoid (particularly in the distal ileum), ulcerating (often confused with an adenocarcinoma) or widely infiltrating.
- Ten to twenty percent are multifocal.
- Seventy percent present with small bowel obstruction (including intussusception), 50% with haemorrhage and a variable number with perforation. Acute symptoms are usually preceded by symptoms of intermittent subacute obstruction for several weeks or months.
- Those not presenting with complications are usually found to have a short history of malaise, anaemia, vague abdom-

inal discomfort, nausea and an abdominal mass. Surprisingly, weight loss is often mild.

- Those with extensive involvement or a partial obstruction may have a malabsorption syndrome with steatorrhoea or a protein-losing enteropathy.
- Spread to the regional lymph nodes occurs early, and distant metastasis occurs to the bone marrow, liver, Waldeyer's ring and CNS.

(b) Investigations

- Routine blood tests may show a mild anaemia and raised LDH level.
- A small bowel enema may show the characteristic 'aneurysmal' dilatation, extrinsic compression, mesenteric mass and often multiple mucosal abnormalities.
- Lesions in the terminal ileum and caecum may be reached and biopsied with a colonoscope.
- An abdominal CT scan and guided biopsy is often possible.
- In many cases, a laparotomy is needed to confirm the diagnosis.

(c) Staging

- Staging procedures include: upper and lower endoscopy, CT scan of the abdomen, frozen-section biopsies at laparotomy, bone marrow biopsy and possibly CSF analysis.
- The same Ann Arbor system of staging as for gastric lymphoma is used.

(d) Treatment

- No consensus has been reached on the therapeutic guidelines for primary small bowel lymphomas.
- For localized, low-grade tumours, surgical resection is the treatment of choice. Chemotherapy and radiotherapy are not effective.
- High-grade lymphomas should also be treated surgically, even if only as a debulking procedure. Chemotherapy is the mainstay of treatment for all high-grade tumours (with or without metastasis). The specific regime depends on the histological type, tumour bulk and extent of spread.

2. Immunoproliferative small intestinal disease (IPSID). This group of lymphomas is thought to derive from a prolonged antigenic stimulus to the gut mucosa (probably by an infectious organism). This is thought to cause proliferation of the enteric immune system in the mucosa and mesenteric lymph nodes. In the majority of cases, an α heavy chain (IgA)-producing B lymphocyte clone develops, earning it the synonym of α-chain disease. The disease is rarely found outside of the following population groups: Arabs and Jews in the

Mediterranean basin, Iranians from southern Iran, and South African black people. Most patients are between 15 and 30 years of age (as compared to western lymphomas) and are of poor socio-economic circumstances.

(a) Characteristic features

- The entire length of the small bowel is thickened by a mixed lymphocyte and plasma cell infiltrate. Nodules or discrete masses are also possible, these being most marked in the duodenum and jejunum (as compared with western lymphomas, where ileocaecal involvement predominates).
- Patients typically present with features of malabsorption and protein-losing enteropathy together with intermittent colicky abdominal pain. Finger clubbing occurs in one-third of cases.

(b) Investigations

- Serum immuno-electrophoresis shows an α heavy chain paraprotein with depressed immunoglobulin levels in 70%.
- Small bowel barium studies and push enteroscopy with jejunal biopsies are needed to confirm the diagnosis.

(c) Treatment

- A prolonged course of tetracycline and metronidazole (*Giardia lamblia* infestation is frequently superimposed) improves the malabsorption syndrome in the early stages and has been known to induce a complete remission.
- Combination chemotherapy is effective in the more advanced stages with autologous bone marrow transplantation an option for selected cases.
- As large areas of the small bowel are involved, surgical resection is usually not possible.
- Most cases follow a relapsing and remitting course and most patients eventually die of their disease (usually from cachexia, infections, perforation or small bowel obstruction).

Further reading

Martin IC, Aldoori MI. Immunoproliferative small intestinal disease: Mediterranean lymphoma and alpha heavy chain disease. *British Journal of Surgery*, 1994; **81(1)**: 20–4.
Thomas CR Jr, Share R. Gastrointestinal lymphomas. *Medical and Pediatric Oncology*, 1991; **19(1)**: 48–60.

Related topics of interest

Coeliac disease (p. 44)
Colonic polyps (p. 52)

Malignant tumours of stomach (p. 195)

ULCERATIVE COLITIS – BACKGROUND AND CLINICAL FEATURES

Background

Ulcerative colitis is an inflammatory condition of the colonic mucosa. The rectum is usually involved, with variable amounts of the more proximal colon affected, from none 'proctitis' (25% of cases, of whom about 25% will eventually develop more proximal disease) to all 'pancolitis' (25% of cases). 50% have disease of the left colon only. Rectal sparing has been described from disease onset; however, this pattern usually results from the use of topical rectal treatments.

Its prevalence is high (50–80 per 100 000) in Northern and Western Europe, USA and Australia, and relatively low elsewhere. It may commence at any age, but most commonly between the ages of 20–40 and 55–70 years. There is no association with gender or social class. Ten to twenty percent of patients will have other family members affected. It is commoner in non-smokers (the reverse of the situation in Crohn's disease) particularly in the first 2 years after stopping smoking.

Aetiology

The cause is unknown. Possible candidates include:

- Infections (certain strains of *E. coli*).
- Food allergies (milk).
- Autoimmune disease.
- Abnormal T-cell and macrophage activation.
- Lack of colonic short-chain fatty acids.
- NSAIDs (these may cause a disease indistinguishable from ulcerative colitis, and can exacerbate existing inflammatory bowel disease (ulcerative colitis or Crohn's)).

Clinical features

Bloody diarrhoea (often with mucus), with or without colicky abdominal pain, is the main symptom. Symptoms are usually present for weeks or months before presentation, but they may be acute and mimic infective colitis (which itself can trigger an attack). Proctitis results in fresh rectal bleeding, tenesmus and faecal incontinence. In proctitis, constipation *can* be prominent.

In severe attacks, systemic symptoms (nausea, malaise, anorexia) are common. Symptom severity usually correlates with disease severity.

Physical signs may include fever, tachycardia, pallor, and tenderness over the involved colon. Young patients may appear deceptively well. Steroids may mask clinical signs, including those of peritonism after bowel perforation.

Investigations may show an iron deficiency anaemia, leucocytosis, thrombocytosis, raised ESR and CRP and hypoalbuminaemia.

Assessment of severity

Truelove and Witts' criteria provide a convenient clinical assessment of disease severity and have stood the test of time:

- Mild disease – less than four stools daily (with or without blood), no systemic symptoms and a normal haemoglobin and ESR.
- Moderate disease – more than four stools daily but with minimal systemic symptoms.
- Severe disease – more than six bloody stools daily with one or more of: fever >37.8 °C, tachycardia >90 bpm, anaemia <10.5 g/dl, ESR >30 mm/hour.

Investigations and diagnosis

- Stool samples should be sent to exclude infective colitis.
- A plain supine abdominal radiograph may show mucosal oedema, small and large bowel dilatation, and mucosal islands in severe disease. Stool is usually absent from regions of actively inflamed mucosa; constipation may be seen proximally.
- Diagnosis may be strongly suggested by appearances at sigmoidoscopy and confirmed by rectal biopsy. Important early differentials are infections, and in older patients malignancy, diverticular disease and bowel ischaemia.
- Biopsies are best taken from the posterior wall within 10 cm of the anal margin to reduce the risk of perforation. Microscopic features include inflammatory cell infiltration confined to the mucosa; crypt abscesses; goblet cell depletion and epithelial ulceration. In chronic cases, crypt distortion, lymphoid aggregation and chronic inflammatory cell infiltration are seen.
- Colonoscopy is not essential during an acute presentation, but appears safe in experienced hands. It is useful in assessing the histological extent of disease (which often exceeds the macroscopic extent), and for cancer surveillance in chronic cases. In long-standing cases the mucosa becomes atrophic and featureless with absent haustral folds, and inflammatory (pseudo-) polyps.
- In mild to moderate disease, in the absence of colonic dilatation, an air-contrast barium enema or single-contrast water-soluble enema may be performed. With active disease, mucosal granularity is seen in mild cases and collar-stud ulcers (which follow the taenia coli) in severe cases.

Differential diagnosis

Crohn's disease, ischaemic colitis, collagenous colitis, infective colitis, pseudomembranous colitis and drug-induced (especially NSAIDs, antbiotics) colitis may all mimic ulcerative colitis on macroscopic grounds. If proctitis only is present, gonococcal or chlamydial infection should be excluded. In the immunocompromised or HIV-infected patient, HSV, CMV or

Table 1. Features of ulcerative colitis and Crohn's colitis

	Ulcerative colitis	Crohn's colitis
Clinical	Bloody diarrhoea	Abdominal mass
		Peri-anal lesions
		Frank bleeding less frequent
Sigmoidoscopy	Rectum 'always' involved	Rectum involved in 50%
Radiology	Extends proximally from rectum	Segmental disease
	Continuous fine mucosal inflammation	Fissures, fistulae, deep ulcers
	Superficial ulceration	Strictures
	Strictures very rare	Small bowel involved
Histology	Acute inflammatory mucosal infiltrate	Transmural lymphocyte infiltrate
	Goblet cell depletion	Goblet cells preserved
	Crypt destruction and distortion	Granulomas characteristic
	Crypt abscesses	

atypical mycobacterial infection should be considered. *Table 1* may help to differentiate ulcerative colitis from Crohn's colitis.

Extra-intestinal manifestations

These occur in 10–20% of cases.

1. Related to the activity of the colitis. These disappear after proctocolectomy.

- Acute large joint oligo-arthropathy (10–15% of patients during an acute attack).
- Erythema nodosum (may be caused by sulphasalazine).
- Episcleritis and anterior uveitis (5–8%).
- Oral aphthous ulcers.
- Pyoderma gangrenosum (uncommon – may persist during remission).

2. Unrelated to the activity of the colitis
- PSC (see p. 238). Patients with ulcerative colitis should have their liver enzymes checked every 6 months, and persistent elevations investigated with ERCP. Cholangiocarcinoma develops in about 5%.
- Ankylosing spondylitis (1–2 %).
- Sacroiliitis.

Further reading

British Society of Gastroenterology. Inflammatory bowel disease. *BSG Guidelines in Gastroenterology*, September 1996.

Forbes A. *Clinicians' Guide to Inflammatory Bowel Disease*. London: Chapman and Hall Medical, 1997.

Hanauer SB. Medical therapy of ulcerative colitis. *Lancet*, 1993; **342**: 412–17.

Hanauer SB. Inflammatory bowel disease. *New England Journal of Medicine*, 1996; **334**: 841–8.

Rampton DS. Ulcerative colitis. *Prescribers Journal*, 1997; **37(4)**: 220–31.

Related topics of interest

ULCERATIVE COLITIS – MEDICAL AND SURGICAL MANAGEMENT

As for Crohn's disease, management of ulcerative colitis should be considered in two phases: treatment of the acute attack to induce remission in new/relapsed disease, and then maintenance of remission.

Treatment of an acute attack

Mild or moderate attacks

Patients who are systematically well with manageable levels of diarrhoea can usually be managed as out-patients. Mild attacks are managed with an oral 5-ASA preparation (see below) and twice-daily steroid retention or foam enemas. Many patients also require oral prednisolone (20–40 mg daily for a month, gradually reducing over the next 1–2 months once remission is achieved).

Proctitis

- Local steroid suppositories, retention or foam enemas (depending on the patient's preference), or local 5-ASA preparations (suppositories, liquid or foam enemas) are equally effective (the latter are more expensive).
- An oral 5-ASA agent is also beneficial in the acute attack and for the maintenance of remission.
- Some cases are very resistant to treatment and oral or i.v. steroids may be needed.
- For severe refractory disease, cyclosporin enemas, oral methotrexate and short-chain fatty acid enemas have been used in specialist centres.
- Proximal constipation is a well-recognized complication of proctitis and should be treated with osmotic laxatives or fibre supplements.
- Surgery is sometimes the best option for very refractory distal disease.

Treatment of severe attacks

Patients with a severe attack present as a medical emergency. The mainstays of treatment are steroids, i.v. fluids, 5-ASA compounds, regular clincial review and liaison with the surgical team to detect toxic megacolon and determine the optimum timing of surgery if required. Important aspects of management include:

- Intravenous hydrocortisone (100 mg every 6 hours) and rectal steroids (twice daily). Rectal steroids are often best tolerated in the form of 100 mg of hydrocortisone in 100 ml of 0.9% saline given over 30 min via an i.v. giving-set. Oral prednisolone (40 mg daily) should be started in place of i.v. hydrocortisone after 5 days, and gradually decreased over the next 8 weeks.

- Fluid and electrolyte balance (particularly potassium levels) should be carefully monitored and corrected. Serum electrolytes, full blood count, CRP and ESR should be checked daily.

- A full-dose 5-ASA agent should be commenced when the patient is able to tolerate oral medication.

- Patients should be examined at least twice daily to assess the temperature, pulse, blood pressure, abdominal girth and tenderness, and a stool chart should be recorded. Abdominal radiographs should be checked daily for signs of acute dilatation (see below), peritoneal free air or ileus.

- Blood cultures should be obtained and a stool specimen collected for microscopy and *C. difficile* toxin assay.

- Intravenous antibiotics (cefuroxime and metronidazole) are administered in most centres; however, their benefit is unproven.

- A blood transfusion is needed if the haemoglobin falls below 10 g/dl.

- The thromboembolism risk is increased in active inflammatory bowel disease. The benefit of subcutaneous heparin as prophylaxis needs to be balanced against the problems of increased colonic blood loss.

- Antidiarrhoeals (e.g. codeine, loperamide), antispasmodics and anticholinergics should be avoided due to the risk of colonic dilatation.

- Oral intake does not affect the outcome; however, most patients are anorectic and sips of fluid are permissible. Furthermore the response to the re-introduction of food may be a useful indicator for the need for colectomy.

- Nutritional supplements are usually needed and total parenteral nutrition will be required for those very sick patients who are poorly nourished or for those likely to need a colectomy.

If the response has been inadequate after 5–7 days, cyclosporin (4 mg/kg daily i.v. then 6–8 mg/kg orally) is used in some specialist centres. It is effective in inducing clinical remission in 60–80% of patients resistant to i.v. steroids; however, the relapse rate is high when it is discontinued. It is associated with a high incidence of serious adverse effects, including hypertension, epilepsy (usually in patients with a low serum magnesium and/or cholesterol), nephrotoxicity, opportunistic infections (including *Pneumocystis carinii* pneumonia), renal impairment, peripheral neuropathy and hypertrichosis.

Indications for surgery

Ulcerative colitis is cured by removal of the colon. Twenty-five percent of patients with a severe attack will require an emergency colectomy. Surgical options include panproctocolectomy with ileo-anal pouch or permanent ileostomy, and rarely subtotal colectomy with ileorectal anastomosis. The decision and timing can be difficult and collaboration between physicians and surgeons is needed. Indicators of a poor prognosis and the probable need for colectomy are:

1. *Within the first 24 hours:*
- More than nine stools/day, or three to eight stools/day with a CRP of >45.
- Tachycardia.
- Temperature >38°C.

2. *Within the first 4 days:*
- Serum albumin <30 g/l.
- Persistently elevated ESR and CRP.
- Abdominal radiograph showing mucosal islands (polypoid areas of mucosal oedema) in the colon and/or three or more loops of distended small bowel.

Complications of acute attacks of ulcerative colitis

1. *Acute dilatation (toxic dilatation/megacolon).* This occurs in 5% of attacks and may be precipitated by hypokalaemia or the injudicious use of opiates or antidiarrhoeals. Apart from the clinical features of severity listed above, such patients also display abdominal distension, high-pitched bowel sounds, peritonism (which may be masked by steroids), and a reduction in bowel movements (which may be misinterpreted as a clinical improvement). The abdominal radiograph shows a dilated transverse colon of >5–6 cm in diameter, and the loss of the haustral pattern. If dilatation is seen at the onset of an acute attack, a joint medical and surgical decision for a trial of medical treatment and close monitoring for 24–48 hours is justified. Failure to improve after this is an indication for urgent colectomy. Acute dilatation which develops during medical treatment is an indication for an emergency colectomy.

2. *Perforation.* This rare complication usually occurs with acute dilatation, but may occur in its absence, or secondary to colonoscopy. Signs of peritonitis may be masked by the use of steroids. An erect abdominal radiograph shows free air under the diaphragm. Aggressive fluid, electrolyte and blood replacement, and i.v. antibiotics (ampicillin, metronidazole and gentamicin) should be followed by emergency colectomy.

Maintenance of remission

Patients with distal disease and a relapse rate of less than once a year probably need no maintenance treatment. The majority of patients require a 5-ASA preparation, and those with frequent relapses should be prescribed azathioprine in addition. Corticosteroids have no role in the maintenance of remission.

Aminosalicylates

Long-term therapy with a 5-ASA agent reduces the relapse rate four fold. The original compound, sulphasalazine, consists of a sulphonamide carrier (sulphapyridine) linked to 5-ASA by an azo bond, which is cleaved by colonic bacteria, releasing the active 5-ASA. The sulphapyridine is absorbed (the main cause of side-effects). Adverse effects occur in 15–20% of patients. These may be dose related (nausea, vomiting, folate malabsorption, headache, alopecia), or non-dose related (fever, hypersensitivity rashes, Heinz-body haemolytic anaemia, aplastic anaemia, agranulocytosis, oligospermia). Male patients should be warned of the risk of infertility, which is reversible on stopping the drug. Newer alternatives (see below) are better tolerated, but are considerably more expensive.

The generic name for enteric-coated or delayed-release preparations of 5-ASA is mesalazine. Newer 5-ASA agents, without the sulphapyridine carrier molecule, are listed below:

- Asacol (5-ASA coated with a resin (Eudragit-S) which dissolves at pH 7 or above, i.e. in the distal ileum and colon).
- Salofalk (resin (Eudragit-L) coated, released at pH 6 – predominantly in the distal jejunum and ileum).
- Pentasa (delayed-release 5-ASA in ethylcellulose microspheres which disintegrate at pH >6, in the small and large bowel).
- Olsalazine (two molecules of 5-ASA linked by an azo bond, cleaved by colonic bacteria. Causes watery diarrhoea in about 5%, more suitable for patients with distal disease).
- Balsalazide (5-ASA is linked via a diazo bond to an inert carrier, cleaved by colonic bacteria. It is likely to have the best colon delivery characteristics and is better tolerated than the other preparations).

Adverse effects of mesalazine are relatively rare (5% of patients). These include gastrointestinal upsets, neutropenia, aplastic anaemia, and interstitial nephritis. All patients should be warned of these symptoms (unexplained bleeding, bruising, sore throat, fever or malaise), and should be monitored with regular full blood counts. Electrolytes should be monitored intermittently (particularly those on Asacol) to detect possible interstitial nephritis.

Mesalazine and sulphasalazine are available as retention enemas/suppositories, suitable for maintenance therapy in disease distal to the splenic flexure/rectum, respectively.

Azathioprine

Azathioprine (2 mg/kg/day) can be used as maintenance therapy and as a steroid-sparing agent in chronic relapsing disease. Up to 6 months of treatment may be needed before it becomes effective. The main adverse effects include nausea, rash, fever and diarrhoea (improved with a gradual introduction, starting at a low dose), and rarely pancreatitis, cholestatic hepatitis and marrow suppression. Blood checks are needed every 2–4 weeks for the first 3 months and then every 1 or 2 months during treatment.

Other maintenance therapies

Unlike Crohn's disease, elemental diets are not effective. Fish oil supplements and short-chain fatty acids have been shown to be beneficial in the short term (although are often poorly tolerated). Other therapies under evaluation include nicotine therapy (as patches or enemas) and anti-tumour necrosis factor antibodies.

Surgery

Outside of treatment of acute attacks, surgery should be considered in the following circumstances:

- Refractory disease (even if localized to the left colon or rectum).
- Complications from/intolerance of medical therapy (especially long-term steroid side-effects).
- Growth retardation in children.
- High-grade dysplasia or malignancy.

The type of surgery will depend on the preferences of the individual patient and surgeon. Total colectomy with preservation of anal sphincters and creation of an ileo-anal pouch anastamosis is one preferred option, leaving a high percentage of patients with acceptable continence without a stoma. A proportion of patients will not be suitable for this surgical option, or will develop complications, and require a proctocolectomy with end ileostomy.

Pouchitis

See topic 'Colitis – non-specific' (p. 50).

Treatment of ulcerative colitis in pregnancy

Pregnancy is not known to exacerbate colitis. Treatment of exacerbations and maintenance therapy are the same in pregnancy as during other times. Corticosteroids and aminosalicylates are safe during pregnancy/breast-feeding. Azathioprine has been inadvertently used in pregnancy with no adverse effects; however, if possible, it is safest to avoid it.

Colonic cancer surveillance

The risk of developing colon cancer correlates with the extent and duration of disease. The risk is maximal for those with pancolitis; those with limited disease (distal to the splenic flexure) do not appear to be at increased risk. The risk is only appreciable in those who have had colitis for more than 10 years. The cumulative risk is approximately 7–15% at 20 years. Despite this, prospective trials of the efficacy of disease prevention by regular colonoscopy have given conflicting results. In practice, individual centres are limited by the local resources and funding.

- Patients with extensive disease, for longer than 10 years, should be considered for a colonoscopy every 2 years. Biopsies should be taken at intervals and from any suspicious site.
- If high-grade dysplasia is found, and confirmed with repeat biopsies, prophylactic colectomy is advised.
- If lesser grades of dysplasia are found, more frequent examinations are needed.

Prognosis and follow-up

The severity, extent, and responsiveness to treatment of ulcerative colitis is very variable: 80% of patients have intermittent attacks; 10–15% have chronic continuous disease; and 5–10% will have a severe initial attack requiring an urgent colectomy. Mortality during an acute attack (including that for acute colectomy) is less than 2%. Most patients have a near normal life expectancy, with acute attacks and colonic cancer being the principal causes of mortality. Quality of life is impaired to some degree in most patients.

Patients with well-controlled distal colitis can be followed up by their general practitioners. Full blood counts, serum electrolytes and liver enzymes should be checked 6–12-monthly. A colonoscopy with biopsies should be performed about 8–10 years after the diagnosis to confirm the extent of disease and for cancer surveillance. Those that relapse should be referred immediately back to the out-patient department.

Those in remission with more extensive ulcerative colitis require follow-up as an out-patient every 6–12 months, with earlier open access in the event of a relapse. Assessment of adequacy and compliance with maintenance treatment is important, as about 70% of patients with untreated disease relapse each year and up to 30% eventually require surgery. Blood tests (as above) should be checked every 6 months and more frequently in active disease. Elevated liver enzymes, in the absence of alcohol consumption or enzyme-inducing medication, should be investigated with an ERCP to exclude primary sclerosing cholangitis. The cancer surveillance strategy outlined above should be followed.

Useful sources of information and support for patients, doctors and carers

- NACC (National Association for Colitis and Crohn's Disease), PO Box 25, St Albans, Hertfordshire AL1 1AB.
- British Digestive Foundation, 3 St Andrew's Place, Regent's Park, London NW1 4LB.
- Ileostomy Association, PO Box 23, Mansfield, Nottinghamshire NG18 4TT.

Further reading

British Society of Gastroenterology. Inflammatory bowel disease. *BSG Guidelines in Gastroenterology*, September 1996.

Forbes A. *Clinicians' Guide to Inflammatory Bowel Disease*. London: Chapman and Hall Medical, 1997.

Hanauer SB. Medical therapy of ulcerative colitis. *Lancet*, 1993; **342**: 412–17.

Hanauer SB. Inflammatory bowel disease. *New England Journal of Medicine*, 1996; **334**: 841–8.

Rampton DS. Ulcerative colitis. *Prescribers Journal*, 1997; **37(4)**: 220–31.

Related topics of interest

WHIPPLE'S DISEASE

Whipple's disease is a rare multiorgan disease, primarily involving the intestinal tract. It is caused by infection with the actinobacterium *Tropheryma whippelii* (Whipple's bacillus). The disease almost exclusively affects Caucasian males between the ages of 40 and 70. The organism is a common soil and water saprophyte, and the disease frequently affects those who work on farms or building sites. It is usually found in central Europe and North America and has rarely been described elsewhere.

Clinical features

Common features at presentation include those of malabsorption (weight loss, diarrhoea, rarely steatorrhoea), anaemia (90%), hypotension, abdominal pains and arthralgias. Symptoms are often non-specific and gastrointestinal features may be absent, making the diagnosis difficult. Other systems involved are:

- Central nervous system (CNS). Ten percent present with neurological symptoms (although pathological evidence of CNS involvement is found in almost all cases). Features include progressive dementia, subtle personality changes, seizures, hemiparesis and ophthalmoplegia. CNS involvement is a frequent cause of long-term morbidity.
- Half of patients have generalized hyperpigmentation which is not associated with adrenal insufficiency.
- Rheumatological. A migratory arthropathy of large joints is common and may precede the other symptoms by several years. Sacroiliitis and spondylitis may occur.
- Cardiovascular. Endocarditis, myocarditis or pericarditis occur rarely, but subclinical signs are found at autopsy in up 50% of cases.
- Renal. Glomerulonephritis, chronic interstitial nephritis and IgA nephritis are described. Sixty percent of patients have abnormalities on urinalysis.
- Eyes. Uveitis, retinitis and ophthalmoplegias may occur.
- Respiratory. Dyspnoea, chronic cough and chest discomfort are common in all cases. Pleurisy, pleural effusions, interstitial pneumonitis and hilar lymphadenopathy are relatively common, but usually only found on post-mortem. The respiratory signs may mimic sarcoidosis.
- Lymphadenopathy. Peripheral lymphadenopathy, hilar lymphadenopathy, and lymphoedema may occur.

Diagnosis

As the organism predominantly affects the proximal small bowel, the diagnosis is made by a biopsy of the distal duodenum. Biopsies show increased numbers of histiocytes within the lamina propria with characteristically foamy, eosinophilic cytoplasm and clear intracytoplasmic inclusions. The cytoplasm is stuffed with dense granular material which is positive on periodic acid–Schiff (PAS) staining, and corresponds to intact or partially degraded bacteria. Electron microscopy will show numerous bacilli engulfed in phagolysosomes within the histiocytes.

Similar clinical and histological features may be seen in patients with AIDS and *Mycobacterium avium* infection. Biopsies should therefore also be stained to exclude acid-fast bacilli.

Treatment   Tetracycline or trimethoprim-sulphamethoxazole for 1 year is the treatment of choice. Neurological disease is the commonest cause of long-term morbidity, and relapses sometimes occur in despite adequate antibacterial treatment. Trimethoprim-sulphamethoxazole may be associated with a lower risk of CNS relapses.

Further reading

MacDermott RP, Graeme-Cook FM. Case records of the Massachusetts General Hospital. *New England Journal of Medicine,* 1997; **337**: 1612–19.

Related topic of interest

Malabsorption (p. 189)

WILSON'S DISEASE

This rare, autosomal recessive condition has a prevalence of 1 in 30 000. The manifestations of the disease are a result of increased copper accumulation, presumably due to reduced biliary excretion, which results in progressive tissue damage. This predominantly affects the liver, basal ganglia of the brain (hence the old term 'hepato-lenticular degeneration'), and leads to the formation of characteristic corneal pigmentation (Kayser–Fleischer rings). The Wilson's disease gene is located on the long arm of chromosome 13; genetic investigation of affected families is possible. The exact metabolic defect causing the disease is unknown.

Clinical features

The disease usually presents between the ages of 5 and 30 and very rarely presents in those over the age of 50. Liver disease usually manifests itself in children and young adults, whilst neuropsychiatric changes become more prominent over the age of 20.

1. Hepatic form. Wilson's disease should be considered in any young patient presenting with acute or chronic liver disease.

- Fulminant hepatitis is characterized by progressive hepatocellular failure (jaundice, ascites, encephalopathy), renal failure and acute intravascular haemolysis. The latter is due to the destruction of erythrocytes by the sudden release of copper from necrotic hepatocytes. This usually occurs in previously healthy children or young adults and Kayser–Fleischer rings and other stigmata of the disease are often absent.
- Chronic hepatitis typically presents between the ages of 10 and 30, with jaundice, elevated liver enzymes and hypergammaglobulinaemia. Neurological manifestations usually develop several years later.
- Cirrhosis may develop insidiously, presenting with signs and symptoms of chronic liver disease. Neurological signs may be absent, even in established liver disease. Unlike some other forms of cirrhosis, the incidence of hepatocellular carcinoma does not appear to be increased.

2. Neuropsychiatric form. The neurological manifestations may be acute and rapidly progressive, but are usually chronic and insidious. Patients usually present in their early twenties with a tremor, difficulty in writing, slurred speech and facial grimacing. The tremor is characteristically coarse ('wing beating') and other features of parkinsonism are also commonly elicited. Two-thirds of patients develop a slow deterioration in their personality which is often missed in the early stages. Dystonic and choreaform movements are also well described and imply irreversible damage.

3. Eye signs. The characteristic Kayser–Fleischer ring is a greenish brown ring of copper-containing pigment deposited in Descemet's membrane at the periphery of the cornea. It may be seen with the naked eye, but a slit-lamp examination is usually needed to detect it. It is commonly found in those with neuropsychiatric manifestations and hence may be absent in children. Prolonged cholestasis and cryptogenic cirrhosis occasionally produce a similar finding. Grey-brown 'sunflower' cataracts are also occasionally seen.

4. Renal manifestations. Copper deposition in the proximal convoluted tubule results in aminoaciduria, phosphaturia and glycosuria. Proximal renal tubular acidosis is frequent and may result in renal calculi.

5. Other manifestations
- Osteoporosis, osteoarthritis, subarticular cysts and pyrophosphate arthropathy (particularly of the spine) are common.
- Gallstones, due to chronic haemolysis, may occur.
- Acute rhabdomyolysis, due to high skeletal muscle copper levels, is described.
- Hypoparathyroidism is also associated.

Investigations

Serum copper and caeruloplasmin levels are usually low. Caeruloplasmin may also be reduced in liver failure (due to failure of synthesis) and in malnutrition. Caeruloplasmin is an acute-phase reactant, and it may be misleadingly raised (or misleadingly 'normal') due to fulminant hepatitis, oestrogen therapy, pregnancy or cholestasis. In almost all cases, 24-hour urinary copper excretion is raised.

Liver enzymes are raised in most of the hepatic forms. In cases of fulminant hepatitis, Wilson's disease is suggested as the aetiological factor where there are inappropriately low serum transaminases and ALP, and a low ALP/bilirubin ratio.

A liver biopsy is important to confirm the increased copper concentration and to assess the extent of liver damage. The quantitative assessment of liver copper is, however, problematic; biopsy samples may become contaminated by high copper levels in the local water supply, and strict control of sterilization techniques and sample storage is important. The copper concentration often differs in different parts of the same liver; increased liver copper levels are also seen in some normal livers and in any form of prolonged cholestasis.

Treatment

D-penicillamine, at a starting dose of 1.5 g daily in divided doses, is the treatment of choice. This chelates copper, allowing an initial increased renal excretion. Improvement is slow and is assessed clinically (fading of Kayser–Fleischer rings, improvement in tremor, speech and cognition), biochemically (a fall in serum free copper (if initially elevated) to <10 µg/dl, and 24-hour urinary copper to <500 µg) and histologically (resolution of active hepatitis on liver biopsy).

Adverse reactions to D-penicillamine occur in about 20% of patients. These include hypersensitivity reactions, proteinuria, skin wrinkling and an SLE-like syndrome. During the initial 6 months of treatment, white cell and platelet counts should be measured and proteinuria should be sought. Trientine is an alternative if penicillamine cannot be tolerated. Patients are also advised to avoid foods high in copper, e.g. mushrooms, liver, chocolate, peanuts, shellfish. After 2 years of successful treatment, a maintenance dose of 0.75–1 g daily is given for life.

Regular measurements of serum and urinary copper levels are important to assess continued improvement and compliance, as fulminant liver failure can occur if penicillamine is stopped suddenly. Liver transplantation is an option for young patients with fulminant liver failure, or those who do not respond to, or are intolerant of, therapy. The disease tends not to recur in the transplanted liver.

Further reading

Yarze JC, Martin P, Munoz SJ et al. Wilson's disease: current status. American Journal of Medicine, 1992; **92**: 643.

Related topics of interest

INDEX

Cholecystitis
  acute, 102, 119
  chronic, 103
  emphysematous, 102
Cholecystojejunostomy, 29
Choledocholithiasis, 106
Cirrhosis, 14, 40, 86, 101, 143, 180, 223, 278
  risk of hepatocellular carcinoma, 150
  transplantation, 254
Cisapride, 64, 95, 131, 179
Clostridium botulinum, 122
Clostridium difficile, 83, 172, 241
  see also Pseudomembranous colitis
Clostridium perfringens, 121, 122
Coeliac disease, 44, 48, 50, 81, 192
Colitis
  collagenous, 50, 266
  fulminant, 242
  ischaemic, 268
  lymphocytic, 50
Colonic
  carcinoma, 53, 55, 62, 77, 82
  familial adenomatous polyposis, 55, 60, 166
  hereditary non-polyposis colorectal cancer, 55, 59
  polyps, 52, 53, 168
  screening, 55, 58, 167, 278
Constipation, 61, 179, 244
Courvoisier's sign, 28
Creon, 37
Crigler–Najjar syndrome, 185
Crohn's disease, 47, 67, 247
  activity index, 70
  differential diagnosis, 71, 120, 124, 244, 266
  extra-intestinal manifestations, 68
  medical and surgical treatment, 73, 259
Cronkite–Canada syndrome, 201, 261
Cryptosporidium, 83, 125, 171, 238
Curling's ulcer, 86, 108
Cushing's ulcer, 86, 108
Cyclospora, 171
Cystic fibrosis, 40
Cytomegalovirus
  gastropathy, 201
  liver, 174

Dermatitis herpetiformis, 44, 47, 261
Descending perineum syndrome, 63, 64, 66
Diabetes
  gastropathy, 79, 81, 92
  secondary to haemochromatosis, 141

Diarrhoea, 40, 50, 67, 76, 81, 209
  bloody, 50, 118, 119, 124, 241, 244, 265
  chronic, 81, 76, 124, 245
  investigation, 82
  nocturnal, 177
  post-gastrectomy, 229
  traveller's, 118
Dieulafoy's lesion, 135, 139
Disaccharidase deficiency, 81
Diverticular disease
  acute, 251
  diverticulosis, 250
  pseudodiverticula, 251
  stricture, 62
Dubin–Johnson syndrome, 180, 185
Dumping syndrome, 230
Duodenum
  carcinoma, 167
  diverticula, 251
  duodenitis, 116
  tumours, 25
  ulcers, 86, 96, 135, 145
Dysentery
  amoebic, 124
  post-dysenteric irritable bowel, 177
  Shigella, 120
Dyspepsia, 92, 109, 230
  non-ulcer, 92, 148
Dysphagia, 22, 93, 98, 130
  causes of, 98, 196, 219

Empyema of gallbladder, 103
Endoscopic retrograde cholangiopancre-
    atography, 28, 29, 32, 35, 106, 107, 184,
    238
Entamoeba histolytica, 124, 171
Enteric adenovirus, 122
Enteric fever, 119
Enteritis, 244
Enterocolitis, 120
ERCP, *see* Endoscopic retrograde
    cholangiopancreatography
Erythema nodosum, 68, 82, 120

Faecal fat measurement, 36, 84, 191
Faecal occult blood, 59
Famciclovir, 160
Familial adenomatous polyposis, 55, 60, 166,
    196
Fatty liver, 1
Ferritin, 142
Fetor hepaticus, 9, 40
Fibrolamellar carcinoma (of liver), 152

Food intolerance, 177
Food poisoning, 121

Gallbladder carcinoma, 31
Gallstone disease, 69, 94, 101
Gamma glutamyl transpeptidase, 3
Gardener's syndrome, 25
Gastric
  adenomas, 167
  cancer, 92, 109, 140, 195, 197
  carcinoids, 209
  leiomyoma, 25
  leiomyosarcomas, 194
  lymphoma, 199, 201
  MALToma, 145, 200
  outlet obstruction, *see* Pyloric stenosis
  polyps, 25
  stasis, 229
  surgery, 229
  tumours, 25
  ulcers, 86, 96, 108, 135
    benign, 109
    malignant, 109
Gastrin, 89, 132, 146, 211
Gastrinoma, 46, 207
Gastritis
  acute, 112
  autoimmune, 112
  bile reflux, 229
  collagenous, 109, 116
  chronic, 113, 145, 195
  eosinophilic, 115
  granulomatous, 115
  hypertrophic (Menetrier's), 116, 201
  lymphocytic, 116
Gastrojejunostomy, 29
Gastro-oesophageal reflux disease (GORD),
  22, 92, 93, 95, 129, 148
Giardia lamblia, 45, 46, 83, 124, 171, 192,
  264
Gilbert's disease, 180, 185
Globus hystericus, 99
Glucagonoma, 213
Gluten-free diet, 46
Gluten-sensitive enteropathy, *see* Coeliac
  disease

Haematemesis, 135, 224
Haematobilia, 136
Haematochezia, 137
Haemochromatosis, 40, 141, 142
Haemolytic uraemic syndrome, 118
Hairy leucoplakia, 169

Heartburn, 129
  see also Gastro-oesophageal reflux disease
Helicobacter pylori, 86, 87, 88, 93, 94, 96, 97,
  145, 147
  eradication, 88, 96, 110, 147, 201
HELLP syndrome, 187
Helminths, 126
Hepatic artery embolization, 153
Hepatic encephalopathy, 9, 11
Hepatic tumours, 150
  benign, 153
  carcinoma, 150
  screening, 161
  transplantation for, 254
Hepatic vein thrombosis, *see* Budd–Chiari
  syndrome
Hepatitis, 8, 162, 164, 165, 174, 180
  chronic autoimmune 19, 20, 40, 254
  liver transplantation for, 254
  lupoid, 20
  viral
    A, 155
    B, 8, 40, 150, 157, 254
    C, 8, 40, 150, 163, 254
    D, 161
    E, 164
    G, 165
Hereditary non-polyposis colorectal carcinoma,
  55, 59
  see also Gardener's syndrome *and* Colonic
Hiatus hernia, 92, 99, 129, 133
Hirschsprung's disease, 62, 63
Histamine (H2) antagonist, 88, 96, 110,
  131
Histoplasmosis, 172
Howell–Jolly bodies, 44
Human immunodeficiency virus (HIV)
  diarrhoea in, 82, 123, 171
  enteropathy, 45, 172
  gut manifestations, 169, 261
  oesophagitis, 130
  pancreatic disease, 175
  sclerosing cholangitis, 238
Hypersplenism, 41
Hypogammaglobulinaemia, 47, 82
Hypolactasia, 46

Indigestion, 92
  see also Dyspepsia
Inflammatory bowel disease, 60, 81
  see also Crohn's disease *and* Ulcerative
  colitis
Insulinoma, 207, 211

Interferon alpha
  in hepatitis A, 159
  in hepatitis C, 164
  in hepatitis D, 162
Iron deficiency anaemia, 56, 68, 109, 115, 127, 201
Irritable bowel syndrome, 61, 62, 81, 95, 176

Jaundice, 155
  hepatic, 180, 184
  obstructive, 106, 180, 184
  prehepatic, 180, 184
Jejunal diverticulosis, 47

Kaposi's sarcoma, 171, 173
Katayama fever, 128
Krukenberg tumour, 197

Lactase deficiency, 81, 84
Lactate dehydrogenase, 3
Lamivudine, 160
Laxatives, 65, 81
  abuse of, 81, 84
Leiomyoma, *see* Gastric *and* Small bowel
Le Veen shunt, 17
Linitis plastica, 195
Linton tube, 227
Lipiodol, 152
Lithotripsy for gallstones, 105
Liver
  abscesses, 106
  amoeba, 124
  biopsy, 41, 143, 184, 234, 239, 279
  Crohn's disease, 69
  failure (acute), 8, 10
  transplantation, 13, 151, 228, 236, 239, 254, 257
  tumours, *see* Hepatic tumours
Loeffler's syndrome, 126
Lundh test meal, 193, 195

Malabsorption, 81, 189
  bile salt, 81, 177, 244
  chronic pancreatitis, 35, 37, 192
  coeliac disease, 40, 191
  Crohn's disease, 69, 191
  post-gastric surgery, 231
  treatment, 193
Mallory–Weiss tear, 135, 139
MALToma, 145, 200
Meckel's diverticulum, 247, 252
Megacolon, 62, 66
Megaoesophagus, 5

Megarectum, 62
Meig's syndrome, 14
Melaena, 135, 250
Melanosis coli, 177
Menetrier's disease, 116, 195, 201
Mesenteric angiography, 249
Microspora infection, 171
Multiple endocrine neoplasia (MEN), 82
  type I, 207, 208, 210, 211
Murphy's sign, 102
Mycobacterium
  M. paratuberculosis in Crohn's disease, 67
  M. tuberculosis, 173

Nausea, 203
Necator americanus, 127
Necrolytic migratory erythema, 213
Nematodes, 127
Neuroendocrine tumours, 207
Nissen fundoplication, 132
Nitrosamines, 196
Non-steroidal anti-inflammatory drugs (NSAIDs)
  colitis, 50, 265
  peptic ulceration, 86, 87, 90, 108, 135, 148

Octreotide, 174, 202, 210, 212, 213, 214
Odynophagia, 98, 130, 216
Oesophageal
  diverticula, 221
  dysmotility, 219
  manometry, 99, 130, 219
  spasm, 219
  varices, 143, 224, 226, 233
Oesophagitis, 98, 130
Oesophagogastroduodenoscopy (OGD), 83, 109
Oesophagus
  Barrett's, 22, 94, 97
  benign oesphageal stricture, 98, 132
  carcinoma of, 22, 215
  irritable, 219
  'nut cracker', 219
  postcricoid web, 99
Oestrogens (in treatment of angiodysplasia), 140
Oncogenes, 56, 196
Oral ulceration, 68, 76, 98, 169

Pancreas
  carcinoma of, 27, 39
Pancreatitis
  acute, 27, 106, 180